Praise for *Sac*

"A learned and path-opening guide to tl. \
as perfectly suited to the present generation as it is to all times and places. You will discover new folds of yourself within its pages."

—Mitch Horowitz, PEN Award–winning author of \
Occult America and *Uncertain Places*

"A magickal journey into the place where we all need to explore—self-love. Whether you're in a relationship or going it on your own, to explore the secrets and divinity through the lens of our sexuality is not only fun, but healing. This book will be your guide."

—Damien Echols, author of *High Magick* and \
coauthor of *Ritual: An Essential Grimoire*

"Are you ready to reclaim your sensuality? Want to sex up your magick? Wish you could tap into your lust for life and manifest your deepest wishes? This is a modern, inclusive, and sex-positive book filled with tarot, ritual, spells, affirmations, and wisdom. Gabriela's writing is down-to-earth and practical—perfect for adepts but also sex magick newbies. With Gabriela's gentle guidance, you can explore your kinks, bring devotional practices into your bedroom, connect to your wild lust, raise your power, and turn your life into something truly magical."

—Theresa Reed, author of *Twist Your Fate:* \
Manifest Success with Astrology and Tarot

"Gabriela Herstik bids you to leave your shame and hang-ups at the door as she escorts you through the magickal power of sensuality and pleasure in her provocative book. With a strong ethical focus on consent and boundaries, Herstik asserts that sacred sexuality begins with the self. Full of insightful journal prompts to assist the reader in evaluating and reflecting on their personal relationship with sexuality, this book also includes many great energy exercises, meditations, and rituals to tap into the powerful currents of magickal hedonism. *Sacred Sex* is a fantastic guide for those looking to explore themselves and spice up their magickal practice regardless of one's gender or sexual orientation."

—Mat Auryn, bestselling author of *Psychic Witch* and *Mastering Magick*

"Gaby's juicy wisdom invites you into a new erotic relationship with yourself, and life. One you've likely always been yearning for."

—Alexandra Roxo, author of *F*ck Like a Goddess*

"A thrilling and densely informative guide to sex magick and sacred sexuality, laying out a number of paths to the Divine Erotic so every reader can find (at least) one that works for them. Herstik is a compassionate and loving guide through these paths, offering everything from history to tarot spreads to affirmations for each step of your journey."

—Cassandra Snow, author of *Queering the Tarot* and coauthor of *Lessons From the Empress*

"With nuance, wit, and a sparkling dedication to the healing powers of self-lust, Herstik offers up historical context, journal prompts, tarot spreads, spells, ritual guides, and interviews with seasoned practitioners to help readers navigate shame and stigma, conjure embodiment, and delve into the deliciously diverse forms of sexual and spiritual expression at our fingertips. *Sacred Sex* deftly undresses the juicy, transformative magick that lies in becoming—as Herstik writes—a priest/ess of your own pleasure."

—Kristen J. Sollée, author of *Witches, Sluts, Feminists*

"Gabriela Herstik brings the magic of sexuality front and center, in what is nothing less than an expertly guided journey of personal transformation. This tome is crammed full of history, myths, and lore surrounding various practices of sacred sexuality, as well as step-by-step exercises, rituals, affirmations, divinations, and practical advice for anyone who wishes to incorporate a healthy sexuality into their spiritual practice. With discussions on boundaries, mindfulness, working with the moon, transgression, sex work, and more, spiritual practitioners both seasoned and new will find much value in these life-affirming pages."

—Storm Faerywolf, author of *The Satyr's Kiss*

"A wonderful permission slip to all who read it. It does what few spiritual or magical books achieve, which is a dissolution of the boundaries between the sacred and the profane, urging readers to both embrace their true sexuality, and discover the sacred within it. It is written with

Gabriela Herstik's unabashed Aquarian authenticity and considerate and practical wisdom. This book will be medicine for many people."

—Jake Kobrin, artist and wizard

"A road map to living deliciously, with focused and intentional lessons on releasing shame and any other blockages that may lie deep within. Gabriela has created a book with exercises, rituals, and affirmations to inspire you to learn, laying the foundations for your very own fulfilling and sustainable self-lust and sex magick practice. The book is inclusive of dating style, sexuality, and gender, supported by interviews with people from all walks of life."

—Baby Reckless, musician, mixed media artist, and occultist

"The profane meets the sacred in this provocative, yet soulful, exploration of magic and personal mystery that will leave you feeling aroused, empowered, and in tune with your body like never before. This is Herstik at her finest, guiding us through the goose-fleshed terrain of sacred sexuality as she weaves a spell with every word."

—Devin Hunter, bestselling author of *Modern Witch*

"An intensely useful and pleasurable introduction to, and practical manual of, individuation and self-empowerment through the use of sexual energies. In medieval times, Ms. Herstik would have surely been burned as a witch for formulating so clearly what has been known to every genuine spiritual tradition but kept forbidden and occult by draconian forces throughout the ages. Today, she instead joyfully burns the flame of erotic enlightenment so that we can literally unite with ourselves, with others, and with the deeper layers of our psyches as well as our bodies."

—Carl Abrahamsson, author of *Resonances*, *Occulture*, *Anton LaVey and the Church of Satan*, and *Source Magic*

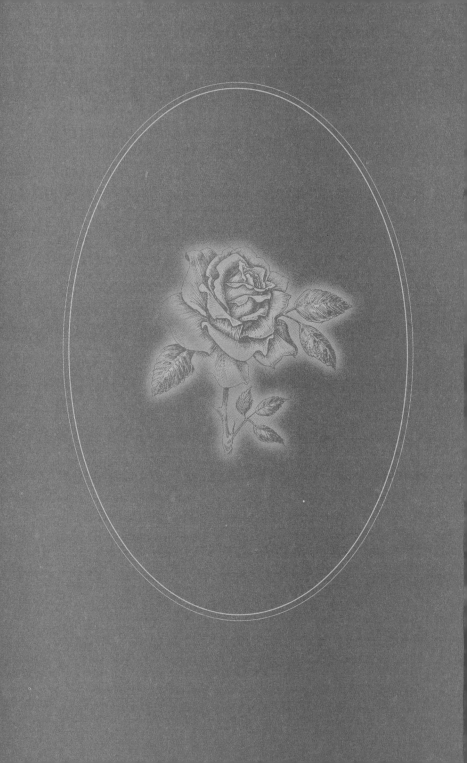

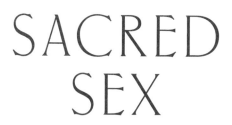

SACRED SEX

The Magick and Path of the Divine Erotic

GABRIELA HERSTIK

A TarcherPerigee Book

tarcherperigee

an imprint of Penguin Random House LLC
penguinrandomhouse.com

Most TarcherPerigee books are available at special quantity discounts for bulk
purchase for sales promotions, premiums, fund-raising, and educational needs.
Special books or book excerpts also can be created to fit specific needs.
For details, write: SpecialMarkets@penguinrandomhouse.com.

Library of Congress Cataloging-in-Publication Data
Names: Herstik, Gabriela, author.
Title: Sacred sex: the magick and path of the divine erotic / by Gabriela Herstik.
Description: 1 Edition. | New York: TarcherPerigee,
Penguin Random House LLC, [2022] | Includes bibliographical references.
Identifiers: LCCN 2022003407 (print) | LCCN 2022003408 (ebook) |
ISBN 9780593421659 (trade paperback) | ISBN 9780593421666 (epub)
Subjects: LCSH: Sex. | Sex—Religious aspects. | Sex customs.
Classification: LCC HQ21 .H447 2022 (print) | LCC HQ21 (ebook) |
DDC 306.7—dc23/eng/20220314
LC record available at https://lccn.loc.gov/2022003407
LC ebook record available at https://lccn.loc.gov/2022003408

Printed in the United States of America
4th Printing

Book design by Laura K. Corless

For Babalon

CONTENTS

CONTENTS

LIST OF MAGICKAL PRACTICES

CHAPTER 1

- Creating a sacred masturbation practice
- Creating a yes/no/maybe list
- Creating an altar for your sacred sexuality
- Consecrating a Sacred Sex Grimoire
- Journal questions
- A tarot spread for understanding your relationship to sacred sex
- Affirmations
- A talisman and amulet spell with the Tower and the Star to release shame and call in sexual sovereignty

CHAPTER 2

- Redefining the erotic
- A condom blessing
- Trauma-informed practices to help you begin reengaging with your sexuality
- Journal questions
- A tarot spread for awakening self-lust
- Affirmations
- A spell to activate self-love and self-lust

CHAPTER 3

- Sex magick 101: the basics

- Sigils and sex magick
- Journal questions
- A tarot spread for diving into the divine erotic
- Affirmations
- A meditation to begin feeling sexual energy in your body
- A sex magick ritual to call forth your fullest sexual potential and power

CHAPTER 4

- A tarot spread for finding your path of sacred sexuality
- Journal questions
- A tarot spread for self-care on the paths of sacred sex
- Affirmations
- A ritual cleansing bath for before or after sacred sex
- Other ways to cleanse yourself before or after sacred sex
- Rituals for energetic sexual hygiene and psychic protection

CHAPTER 5

- Ways to walk the alchemical path
- Journal questions
- A tarot spread for walking through the fire
- Affirmations
- Liber 69: a solar and lunar invocation and ritual of the alchemical marriage

CHAPTER 6

- Journal questions
- A tarot spread for radiating Divine Love into the world
- Affirmations
- A consecration ritual of Divine Union

CHAPTER 7

- Turning orgasms into offerings
- Sex magick through the chakras
- Journal questions
- A tarot spread for arousing erotic devotion
- Affirmations
- Creating a sacred sex devotional

CHAPTER 8

- How to integrate kink into sex magick
- Journal questions
- A tarot spread for embracing the path of the Dark God/dess
- Affirmations
- A sacred S/M ritual with the Devil card for embodying your Divine Deviance

CHAPTER 9

- Journal questions
- A tarot spread for activating the Divine Embodied Masculine
- Affirmations
- A spell to banish toxic masculinity and invoke the embodied and erotic Divine Masculine

CHAPTER 10

- A ritual for cleansing, consecrating, and dedicating clothing and accessories for sacred sex
- Journal questions
- A tarot spread for erotic embodiment in body, mind, and spirit
- Affirmations
- A glamour ritual of body and flesh inspired by Inanna's descent

I

The
Not-So-Basic
Basics

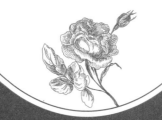

CHAPTER 1

Into the World of Sacred Sexuality

The heart blooms with each breath like a many-petaled rose unfurling. Beneath it, a fire rages with passions of lifetimes, initiation through pain and pleasure—a transmutation of the subtle senses fortified by the power of the Divine Erotic. The body transforms into a temple, as if to welcome the numinous through the flesh. This is sacred sex. This is the esoteric erotic. This is the path of sanctified subversion.

Sacred sexuality. Even reading those words can incite a response. Maybe you rolled your eyes because the phrase feels overhyped and overused. Maybe they kindled a sense of inner knowing that recognizes the juxtaposition as a resonant truth. Maybe you're somewhere in the middle, cautious yet optimistic, worried that this book will be watered-down tantric eye-gazing. Sacred sexuality is many things and spans many cultures and traditions, and like any spiritual or magickal practice, your personal experience will shape how you define it. But if there's one true thing, it's this: conscious, mystical, and devoted connection to your sexuality—the decision to make it sacred—has the power to transform your life.

In the context of this book, you can think of sacred sexuality as a spiritual philosophy and practice rooted in conscious pleasure, and connection to the sexual self as a path to inner wisdom, magick, and evolution. Sacred sexuality is communion with your erotic essence, your sexual sovereignty, your desires, and the well of intuition and soul-expanding medicine within you. It is a way to make sexuality a central part of your spiritual practice. The Divine Erotic is the living current of sexuality that permeates all the universe. It is sacred sexuality embodied as a living force that you have infinite access to. Sacred sexuality is becoming a Priest/ess of your own pleasure, of cultivating and stoking this fire, whether that's with a partner, with partners, or by yourself.

No matter how much society wants you to believe otherwise, sacred sexuality isn't something external. It's not something that only happens when you're in a relationship or partnership, either. Sacred sexuality is your connection to the ecstatic state of transcendent awareness and bliss within. It's your unyielding ability to work with sexual energy to change your world, your heart, and your life. Sacred sexuality is your connection to the carnal self. It's your sacred and subversive discipline, your own inner sex God/dess that's just waiting to be unleashed, and it's the way which you choose to share this with others.

My teachings may differ from others in part because I completely and totally believe that your relationship with sacred sexuality and sacred sex starts within. It's in thinking that you're dependent on anyone else that you may lose the full potential of your erotic power. Even if you're in a relationship, or married, or seriously seeing someone or someones, it all starts with you. It's yours. It belongs to absolutely no one else. And it's in taking the time to honor your desires, to fan the fire of your own flame, to find devotion to yourself, that you can show up to your partner(s) as your fullest sensual self. Sacred sexuality may mean embodying erotic archetypes, accessing ecstatic dimensions, creating rituals around self-love and pleasure, or practicing sex magick. It may be devotion to God/dess. It may mean kink and the taboo, or reading erotic stories, or using adornment and glamour. It may mean working with masturbation or partnered sex. It may look like a conscious unwiring of shame around sex, around seeing yourself as a sexual being or as someone who loves sex. As Cady Heron says in *Mean Girls*, "the limit does not exist."

You can start exactly as you are, right now. You can be single, dating, newly married, married for more than fifty years, widowed, divorced, polyamorous, in an open relationship, or a relationship anarchist. You can be genderqueer, nonbinary, straight, bisexual, intersex, gay, lesbian, or aromantic. You can be Christian, Jewish, atheist, pagan, polytheist, Hindu, or Buddhist. You can be able-bodied or disabled. You can be none of these things or many of these things. You are here, and you are welcome. At its core, sexuality stands apart from any dogma, any religion, and anything prescriptive. It's central to the human experience, not only because it's how we continue the lineage of our species, but because it's something we share access to. Sex is the most primal method we have of consciously connecting with another, and with ourselves.

If you're still unsure of what I mean by "sacred sexuality," here are some of the ways I define it. Feel free to add your own definitions and musings to this list. Sacred sexuality is . . .

- An erotic and esoteric philosophy that honors pleasure as a path to self-knowledge, immanence, expansion, and evolution.
- A way to reclaim your power through erotic magick.
- A personal relationship with your sexual power, first and foremost.
- A way of integrating your sexuality into your spiritual practice and path.

- A means for using sexual energy to shape the reality around you through spells, ritual, and magick.

While sacred sexuality is the seeking of the Divine Erotic, or the highest aspect of the erotic self, sacred sex is the practice. Sacred sex is the act of sharing your sexuality with yourself or with another or with others. It is when you internalize the erotic for the purpose of expansion, gnosis (self-realized knowledge or communion with the Divine), evolution, manifestation, magick, or simply pleasure. It is the art of bringing sacred sexuality into being. It doesn't happen through the mind, but actively through the body, heart, and soul. Practicing sacred sex, whether it's solo or partnered, requires intimacy with the self, first and foremost. It requires vulnerability and communication around limits, desires, and fears. It requires active consent, and a willingness to reach for the erotic edge. It is open and available to all who are willing, but its alchemical furnace is bound to get hot—so hot that it will break down your preconceived notions of who you are and what you want. Slowly, it also will build you back up, transformed, transmuted of all that shit you no longer need and maybe never did. Sacred sex is erotic death and rebirth, leaving you stronger than when you began—and a hell of a lot sexier, too.

In case you're still like "What the fuck is this witch talking about?" here are some of the ways I define sacred sex. Sacred sex is . . .

- Conscious and intentional union for the purpose of transformation, magick, gnosis, and ecstasy.
- The act of sharing your sexuality with the self, partner, beloved, or the whole damn world.
- Bringing spiritual awareness to the erotic.
- Making love to the universe.

- Creating a circuit of sexual energy that you can channel for an intention or purpose.
- A rewriting of society's definition of sex, and the spiritual/occult communities that view polarity between a penis and vagina as necessary for sacramental sex.

Through the two parts of this book, you will be led to a deeper understanding of your sexuality and what makes it so damn sacred. First, we will unwind what sacred sexuality is, how it's been woven through cultures and history, and how this relates to the practice of sex magick, or using sexual energy to cause a change in the material realm. We'll release personal limitations and beliefs, not to mention shame and guilt that you may or may not be conscious of. And you will gain a more expansive understanding of sex through up-to-date sex education.

In the second part, we'll discuss the paths of sacred sex, as well as ways to prepare for them, while keeping in mind that your very sacred, very personal journey may be a combination of several or even one of your own making. And because each chapter is adaptable for your relationship status—whether single, monogamous, polyamorous, or a relationship anarchist—you can come back to them again and again as your circumstances change. The first few rituals are for you alone, to set a foundation for your practice, but nearly all the others are adaptable for solo or partnered exploration (and if they're meant for solo practice, I will include a note to let you know).

Throughout, you will find spells, rituals, journal questions, affirmations, and archetypal inspiration via the wisdom of the tarot to help you understand your multifaceted and mystic sexuality. This book is also peppered with interviews I conducted with sex therapists, astrologers, sexperts, sex workers, erotic artists, and others to bring a more informed and nuanced approach to the world of sacred sexuality. I hope these prompts and conversations spark your exploration so you can develop a practice devoted to your sexuality as it is in each moment. A big part of this is releasing the idea that spending time with your erotic self is frivolous, or wrong, or bad. It also means breaking free of the conditioning that makes you believe that pleasure is only something you can offer partners, not yourself. Whether you've been told that your sexuality is shameful or beautiful is irrelevant because *you* get to decide which stories stay. Sacred sex invites more love and lust into all aspects of your life, which, combined with personal knowing or gnosis, is not only extremely liberating but also has the potential to infuse your entire being with the power of the Divine Erotic.

Not only that, sex doesn't have to look a certain way to be spiritual or even worthwhile. You can explore it casually, or recreationally, or as part of your work. Your ideal may be based in the flesh and not spiritual at all, and that's incredible. Sex positivity means supporting the decisions we all make, whether that's one-night stands, or only having sex in a relationship, or complete abstinence. As long as sex is between consenting adults, it's fair game. *It's your own relationship to sexuality that makes it sacred.*

I bring this up because it can be easy to get on a high horse with spiritual practice, to judge someone else's morals or beliefs based on your own, especially when it comes to something you care about. When you learn something about yourself, you want others to learn the same thing to help themselves. If you find the lessons here transformative and want others to know about this life-changing path, my biggest piece of advice is to simply live it. Be vulnerable and courageous, and lead through example. Shining as the radiant slice of sexiness you are will be infinitely more powerful than trying to convince someone else of what is true for you. When you're authentic and honest around sexuality and self-expression, you invite others to be the same. If they're meant to be on this path, too, they'll find it.

HOW DID WE GET HERE?

Sacred sexuality isn't some twenty-first-century notion. In fact, the idea of sex as a sacred act, the idea of sexuality as a sacred path, spans millennia. It shows up in Kabbalah, mystic Christianity, Sufism, Buddhist and Hindu tantra, alchemy, ceremonial magick, and Goddess worship, among other traditions. The overlap of the erotic and ecstatic also comes from traditions of paganism and witchcraft that centered the experiences of the flesh and worked with the cyclical nature of the earth and self to celebrate the mysteries of sex and death. My hope is that by seeing the ways sexuality and spirituality overlap in different traditions, you'll be able to come to your own conclusions about the potency of combining them, and that by turning to your own culture, religion, and beliefs, you'll create a nourishing spiritual and erotic practice, as people have done for thousands of years.

KABBALAH

Kabbalah is the mystical sect of Judaism that came into being between the thirteenth and seventeenth centuries (and which differs from Hermetic Qabalah, spelled with a Q, though Qabalah's roots are still in mystic Judaism). In Judaism, one of the sacred tenets or sacred deeds, known as a mitzvah, that a married couple can perform is sex. In the Zohar, one of the chief texts in Kabbalah, it is said—in gendered and dated terms—that through sexual union with his beloved, the husband is able to draw down the Godhead; his beloved becomes the feminine face of God, the Shekinah, as he becomes the God. And in case that's too abstract, it also says that this divine and spiritual power exists within a drop of semen. Another example of eroticism in the Jewish scriptures is the Song of Songs, also known as the Song of Solomon, which includes the lines "Let me climb the palm, Let me take hold of its branches; Let your breasts be like clusters of grapes, Your breath like the fragrance of apples" and "How sweet is your love, My own, my bride! How much more delightful your love is than wine, Your ointments more fragrant Than any spice!"

HINDU TANTRA

Tantra, which most likely began in the first millennium CE, spans Buddhism, Hinduism, and Jainism. Etymologically, *tantra* means "to stretch" or "to weave," and you can think of it as "that which expands understanding," a system of knowledge-seeking through the realm of the self, while also seeing the realm of the self as the realm of the Divine.

There are many schools of tantra, and they can be divided into the Left Hand Path (LHP) and the Right Hand Path (RHP). LHP tantra takes the idea of sexual union literally (called maithuna), whereas RHP tantra sees sex and ecstatic union as a metaphor for union with the Divine. For those who practice LHP tantra, the idea of the sacred and taboo are intrinsically related, so by doing what's considered transgressive—like, in parts of Indian society, eating beef or certain grains, drinking wine, or having sex with someone from another caste—you see that everything is everything, and even the most unholy things are holy.

One of the goals of tantra is to activate Shakti and Shiva, or the emanations of the Divine Feminine/creative power and Divine Masculine/consciousness, respectively. The life force within the body is referred to as Kundalini energy, which practitioners envision as a coiled serpent, representing Shakti, that lies at the base of the spine, or the root chakra. One of the aims of tantra is awakening, done by working with and transmuting sexual energy, when this coiled snake stretches out and climbs the energy centers aligned with the spinal column to reach the crown of the head, which represents the potential for fully arousing Shiva, or Divine consciousness.

TAO

Tao, also spelled Dao, is a Chinese philosophy that means "the way." Tao is both a spiritual path and, in the case of cosmic Tao, a belief in the inherent consciousness of all existence. Tao is all about contradictions, as well as unity of the yin and yang. Whereas yin may be considered the feminine aspect of all life, embodied as the Moon, as moist and cold and dark, yang is the masculine, the Sun, light, and heat. Tao makes up the invisible and visible worlds as well as the human personality. Tao is both the thing itself and the practice—a divine juxtaposition of the immaterial.

Taoists focus their gaze on their inner nature through seeking vital energy known as chi, which is stored in the body through energetic reservoirs known as elixir fields. Drawing or collecting chi into the body leads to transformation and cultivation of the self, and one way alchemical practitioners do this is through sexual energy, transforming "sexual essence into spiritual illumination." This is done through practices like the microcosmic orbit, which runs sexual energy up the spine and down through the front of the body, then up the back of the body, creating a loop.

VAJRAYANA: TANTRIC TIBETAN BUDDHISM

Within this synthesis of Buddhism and Bon, or the indigenous teachings of Tibet, everything is seen as emptiness, even matter or form. By cultivating a state of bliss and then contemplating that void, the yogi slowly peels themselves away from the world of the illusion. By sending energy up the spine, through what's called the "secret channel," they generate stillness, presence, and pure-mindedness. Through specific meditations, the practitioner raises energies that correlate to the sexual and spiritual essence of the mother (red drops) and the father (white drops), and when they join, bliss ensues. Vajrayana, like Hindu tantra, requires a close relationship with a guru or spiritual teacher, and the sexual aspects of tantra are shared only with those who have received initiation.

GNOSTICISM

Gnosticism, like tantra, isn't a singular sect but many branches of Christianity that were seen as heretical and were intentionally stamped out between the first and fifth centuries CE. The Gnostics believed that everyone is of the Divine, that everyone is the Divine, but that this has been forgotten in the hazy landscape and illusion of the material world and can only be remembered by personal connection and relationship with the Godhead, known as gnosis. It is through gnosis that you can experience the Divine union of the soul and its counterpart, Sophia, the feminine face of God that means "wisdom." The goal of this mystical path is to free yourself from the bond of matter so you can return to the spiritual realm. The Gnostics let women preach and lead, which was a big turnoff for the Church, and in this way, they were forerunners of many of today's spiritual communities that don't discriminate by gender. You might have heard that Gnostics consumed sexual fluids and had orgies, but the truth is that many Gnostics saw the physical body as a prison, as something to be ignored. Those lingering rumors are based in the Church's fears of unbridled sexual power.

All this is to say that you don't need to follow any specific form of sexual alchemy or magick to connect with your sacred sexuality. All you need is to believe in your own unyielding power. One of the ways you can be reminded of this—and live this—is through archetypes.

THE EROTIC POWER OF THE ARCHETYPE

Throughout this book, we will discuss the evocation of different archetypal powers. By inviting in or embracing archetypal energies, you're more easily able to connect to those aspects of yourself because the archetype is already built into the psyche. Early twentieth-century psychoanalyst Carl Jung coined the term *archetype* to describe themes and concepts that hold universal appeal for all humanity. Archetypes reside in the collective unconscious. Just as we all have conscious and unconscious sides, which can be thought of as the awakened and latent aspects of the self, respectively, so is this played out on a communal scale. The collective unconscious contains common fears, tropes, symbols, and images that hold power because of the way they relate to humanity as a whole. They show up in dreams, art, religion, literature, and film: the superhero who saves the world, the bad girl, the God, the virgin, the whore, the sexpot, etc. Even animals or Gods can become archetypes when what they represent transcends the boundaries of their individual nature.

Working with archetypes is important for all magickal and spiritual practitioners because it allows you to transcend your own experiences and tap into something larger than the self. In this way, you're not limited by your own worldview. If you're doing a ritual for strength and power, you can call on the lion or the Egyptian lion-headed Goddess Sekhmet. If you're sitting in a practice of presence and stillness, you can connect to the archetypal energy of the Buddha, following the path of those who have done this before you and have cleared the way.

Because the erotic and sexual are so ingrained in individual experience, archetypes are a powerful way to move past any limitations that are keeping you stuck. Sacred sexuality is evolving sexuality. It bursts you open to experiences and perspectives that are greater than you—and often unfamiliar to you. Erotic archetypes offer a way to a sexuality that is innately connected to spirit, to something that surpasses the individual. Think of them as blueprints to experiencing the sexual multitudes within.

Society feeds us so many contradictory and dizzying messages about sex, it can obscure our own values or morals. Taking a step back and examining your archetypal power can remind you that sexuality is a facet of your spirituality, and that like your spiritual practice, your sexual and erotic nature isn't static but ever-transforming. Sacred sexuality isn't a journey defined by the destination. Just as your preferences have probably changed—and will continue to change—since you began having sex, so will your relationship with sacred sex change. Working with archetypes is one piece of this puzzle that can help you figure out what feels right for you right now.

THE ARCHETYPAL POWER OF THE TAROT

Another way archetypes present themselves is through the mirror of the tarot. The tarot is a deck consisting of seventy-eight cards, divided into four suites and two arcanas (coming from the Latin *arcanum*, meaning "secret" or "mystery") known as the major and minor arcana, and the court cards. The tarot most likely originated in Italy in the fifteenth century as a deck of playing cards, although some argue it originated in Egypt long before that. What makes a deck a tarot deck is its structure. There are twenty-two cards in the major arcana, each representing major life milestones and the evolution of the human spirit. The forty minor arcana cards are divided into four suits—wands, cups, swords, and pentacles—with an ace through ten in each. Lastly, the sixteen court cards include pages, knights, kings, and queens, although these are sometimes called daughters, sons, mothers, and fathers, or princesses, princes, queens, and kings. The minor arcana cards represent the trials and tribulations you move through in your day-to-day experience, and the court cards represent the people or energies you are being called to connect with over the course of your life. These seventy-eight cards hold up a mirror to the energy of a given situation and can be used for divination (predicting or understanding the future), spell work, meditation, and rituals. The tarot draws a map back into the self and the present moment. It can be a powerful portal to view your experiences in a new light.

Every card in a tarot deck has symbolic meaning, but we'll focus on the major arcana. The tarot speaks in symbols and, thus, in archetypes, and it's in the twenty-two cards of the major arcana that you are able to see the journey of human existence reflected in the collective unconscious. This includes birth, transformation, ego death, trials and tribulations, spiritual reckoning, and self-actualization. The major arcana cards activate internal energies that resonate with their artistic expression. Whether you're contemplating the Empress, the Hierophant, the Lovers, Judgment, or Justice, the symbols here go way beyond the individual, which means the tarot has a vast potential for connecting to universal messages, spiritually and erotically.

In each chapter, I will share the tarot card that best resonates with its themes, rituals, and practices to help you find your own links to its archetypal powers. Having a tarot deck for yourself will come in handy (the Smith-Waite deck is a classic; I've also listed erotic and sexual decks on pages 326–27), but it's not necessary. If you have internet access, you can look up images of the cards, although again, this isn't necessary. The point of sharing the tarot is to help you gaze through a window to a new perspective. Even if you already work with tarot, you probably don't normally view the cards as erotic (and if you do, hello, you are my people). But that's exactly what we're doing here: inviting you into new sexual possibilities, based on energies you have nestled within you, even if you don't recognize or feel them yet. Each chapter is guided by an erotic archetype so you have a framework you can dive into. And because the tarot has so many uses, from artistic inspiration to intonation of its associated Hebrew letter, it can be used as a stepping-stone in your own sacred sex experience based on your personal spiritual practice.

The Magician, who represents working with our will to create change on the material plane, turns into the Sex Magician, who uses ecstasy, orgasm, and sexual energy to transform the physical world. The Hierophant, who shares the exoteric teachings and blessings of religion or spirituality, becomes the erotic votary, guiding you through the sexual mysteries that the ancient priestesses shared at the temples of the Goddesses of Love. The Emperor goes from representing hierarchy and power to being a vessel for the grounded and Divine Masculine, fertile with all possibilities of life and potent with Big Dick Energy. If you don't know anything about the tarot, that's totally okay, and you'll be able to connect with these archetypal powers regardless.

FIRST THINGS FIRST, LET'S GET RID OF SHAME

One of the main tenets I invite you to consider around sacred sexuality aligns with my views around the spiritual in general: your relationship with sacred sexuality is intensely personal. Your sexuality and the way you practice sacred sex depend on *you*. That is worth celebrating! But often, before you get to this place of fully owning and revering your desires, you have to let go of the beliefs and values that you didn't choose for yourself, that culture and family chose for you. This is big work—huge work—and it's one of the foundational aspects of living a liberated life that I will be coming back to again and again.

Later in this chapter, you will find a ritual to help you cut through these cords of shame and guilt. But the first step is having plenty of self-compassion. You haven't done anything wrong and aren't doing anything wrong by wanting to reframe your relationship to sexuality. Self-compassion means treating yourself with care and support like you'd treat your beloved, a best friend, your inner child, or a pet. It's all about being gentle and kind. You are doing the hard work of choosing a new way forward. This may bring up some rough stuff, whether that's past traumas, guilt, or fear, which is normal. Breathe as you go, don't rush the process, and reach out to a friend or therapist as needed.

Another aspect of self-compassion is nonjudgment. If an intense feeling like panic comes up, try your best not to get upset with yourself. Instead, observe your feelings and allow them to move through you. Sometimes this means taking a walk in the sunshine or jumping up and down as you shake your whole body and groan. Sometimes it means a nice long cry, calling your therapist or BFF, taking a salt bath, or practicing yoga or kickboxing. Sometimes it means putting the book down until you're ready to pick it back up. Basically, find a way to be present in your emotion, and let it out through some sort of physical activity or moment of mindfulness. Staying in the moment and not judging your emotional response is a big part of letting your body do its thing without getting stuck in a cycle or story, clearing the way for other emotions to eventually take its place. By moving through these feelings, you allow your body the gift of doing what it needs to do, without stopping or numbing it.

Self-compassion is key because it takes plenty to release the shame and guilt that's been thrust on us around all things sexual and erotic, especially because so many of these messages contradict one another. In her potent, easy-to-read, and informative book *Come as You Are*, sex educator Emily Nagoski shares three messages around sexuality that you likely grew up with: the media message, the medical message, and the moral message.

The media message says, "You are inadequate," and unless you have done everything sexual under the sun—group sex, anal, one-night stands, earth-shattering orgasms—you're a prude.

Meanwhile, the medical message says, "You are diseased," and that sex leads only to diseases, infections, and unwanted pregnancies and that the only kind of sex allowed is missionary and between a man and woman.

The moral message is probably the most pervasive and says, "Sex isn't for you at all but for your partner," and that any exploration before marriage is a sin leading straight to hell. It says sexuality is profane, not at all sacred.

Untangling the messages you've received from society, from your family, and from your religious upbringing is vital. I won't tell you it's easy. The shame will come up in waves, and it's always a bitch to get through, but I can promise you the more you do it, the easier it will get.

Erasing the Duality of Sacred and Profane

One of the things living as an erotic mystic will teach you is that there is no difference between the sacred and profane. In a conversation with my rabbi father—who has been a rabbi in the reform sect of Judaism for nearly forty-five years—he mentioned that the word *profane* only meant "something outside of the temple." Society has distorted this to mean "dirty" or "impure." But when you see yourself as a living temple, as a materialization of the numinous, everything becomes sacred, even sex, and even that which may seem profane to others. Living a life devoted to sacred sex means dissolving this duality and reveling in the holiness of the corporeal.

REFRAMING YOUR RELATIONSHIP WITH SEXUALITY

One of the biggest hurdles to embodying your sacred sexuality is reframing your relationship with this part of yourself. This is a work in progress—a journey, not a destination—and no matter how liberated, confident, slutty, and sex positive you are, it must be revisited again and again. The initial reframing and deprogramming is the hardest, but shame, guilt, and embarrassment will visit you at unexpected and inconvenient times. Each time these feelings emerge, however, the less power they hold over you, the easier it is to move past them, and the less of a struggle it is to step back into your erotic power. You don't have to put pressure on yourself to get it "right" or to wish for sexual liberation and expect to be there. This is a winding road, with adventures around each twist and turn, but each day you show up and decide to embrace your sexual essence, the farther along you are on the way to living your erotic truth.

Remember that you are more than your thoughts or feelings about your sexuality. You are more than your limiting beliefs around what it means to be a sexual being. All the programming around being not enough, too little, too much, is just that—programming. And you have the power to delete that code, and replace it with something more valuable, supportive, and sexy. Your sexuality is powerful and numinous. It's Divine. And you are *allowed to want it. You are allowed to want sex and to want to make it a point of your spirituality and magick.*

RELEASING SHAME THROUGH
THE TOWER AND THE STAR

Two symbols you can use to transform your sexuality are the sixteenth and seventeenth keys (or major arcana cards) of the tarot. In the deck, the sixteenth key is the Tower, which many practitioners are afraid to see in a reading. I get it—this card can seem scary. In the classic Smith-Waite deck, it is a tower that's been struck by lightning, with figures leaping from it, presumably to their death. There is what looks like fire raining down (it's actually the Hebrew letter Yod, the first letter in the Divine four-fold name of God), and gray clouds of smoke against a black background. At the top of the tower, a golden crown is being displaced.

The Tower is intense—but it doesn't have to be scary. It represents the removal of the false crown, or taking away power from that which is unworthy. It represents a sense of destruction at a foundational level, one that calls for a sense of radical honesty with what's necessary and what's not. On one hand, the Tower represents the destruction of negative ego, moving from a place of control and fear to one of surrender and dissolution of the conscious self. For our purposes, the Tower represents your destructive and negative beliefs around sexuality. It represents all the messaging you've picked up that has been holding you back from your power, that has forced you to give it away, whether to partners who you believe deserve pleasure more than you do, to religious institutions who have shamed you, or to family values that have instilled a sense of fear and guilt around sexual expression. The Tower is hierarchical and shows authoritarian powers coming to an end. Whatever you've been giving authority to that doesn't serve you has taken its toll, and now the powers that be—aka the powers within *you*—are destroying it.

Astrologically, the Tower is a correspondent to the planet Mars. Host of the *Bad Astrologers* podcast and astrologer extraordinaire Amelia Quint explains this energy as "the pursuit, sexuality, the visceral, and sexual chemistry." Mars is the warrior planet, the planet of aggression and power, the sexual destruction to Venus's erotic creation. How appropriate that through the erotic archetype of the Tower, you can use Martian energy to rescind the beliefs keeping you from living the wildly delicious sex life of your dreams. When you are working against Martian energy, this can feel like the Tower itself, teetering closely to total collapse. But when you channel and hone this as a chance for intentional destruction of old systems of belief, it tells you not to reject your carnal love and lust but to *embody* it. What beliefs around sex and spirituality have been slowly destroying your connection to yourself? How can you decimate them and take back your power?

Without the pain and anguish of the Tower, we wouldn't reach the Star, the seventeenth key of the tarot that follows the carnage of Martian energy. The Star is one of the most auspicious cards of the deck, featuring a nude figure pouring two jugs of water, one into a stream or river and one onto land that then turns into tributaries. Above her shine eight-rayed stars. The Star is an omen of cosmic guidance, of coming back to a sense of grounded mysticism, of spiritual power. The Star is balance of inner and outer wisdom. It represents the potential for transformation that happens when you allow your limiting beliefs to be uprooted and sacrificed. It is when you are connected to your inner sex God/dess, your inner sex mystic, your inner sex witch, that this inner knowing can guide you toward expansion, transcendence, pleasure, and understanding of self. Your sexuality is the guiding star, and you just have to orient yourself under its rays. You may start your journey under the energy of the Tower, but by the end of this book, you will be the Star.

*At the end of this chapter, you will be guided in
working with the Tower and the Star to create an amulet
to banish negative beliefs around sex and a talisman
to draw in supportive beliefs instead.*

THE TOOLS OF SACRED SEXUALITY

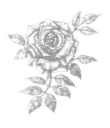

Sacred sexuality is one way of gaining awareness of the erotic within the self, but the path itself is as diverse as each mystic who walks it. And what is the point of sex and sexuality in general if it doesn't feel good to *you*? It's about turning on your heart, your soul, and your spirit. Pleasure is one of the guiding principles here because pleasure, in its most ecstatic and connected forms, has the potential to blur boundaries between the self and the other. One of the perks of sacred sex is that your definition of pleasure will evolve past penetration itself, into anything that touches you in a way that feels cosmic, delicious, and far-reaching. There's not one way to get here, either. It takes devotion, and if there's something to be devoted to, why not make it the pursuit of pleasure? Being a Priest/ess of Erotic Devotion means you are not only committed to the discovery of your sexual essence, but that you live it.

The tools we will touch on the most are the ones I personally have felt transformed by. I encourage you to come up with your own, and to dedicate time to exploring and uncovering them. Keeping a grimoire, a magickal diary strictly for the exploration of the erotic, will serve you well if you decide to be the sex sorcerer/sorceress of your dreams. That way, you have a record of the tools you used, the rituals you worked with, and what resonates and what doesn't, which makes it much easier to look back and track your growth over time. There is a ritual for creating a Sacred Sex Grimoire at the end of this chapter.

The following practices are the foundation for the rest of this book, and we will discuss them more deeply as we continue on this journey together.

Energy work and awareness. Energy is everything, and everything is energy. Even though you seem to be living in a material world, if you were to zoom in to the atoms making up everything, they would mostly just be space, and they wouldn't be solid at all, but vibrating. Energy can be neither created nor destroyed, simply recycled and reused, so when you are working with energy, you are working with what has made up everything in the universe since the beginning of time. Energy work is a bedrock of sacred sexuality. I'm not talking about energy healing like reiki or acupuncture or massage, but *manipulating and moving energy through the channels of the subtle body as a means of raising and connecting with sexual energy.* Energy moves through our bodies in what are known as nadis in yogic tradition, meridians in Chinese medicine, and channels in Buddhism. These channels move through the etheric body, which is the part of the spiritual body most connected to the physical body.

When you are practicing sex magick, or working with sex for a purpose, you will be drawing this energy through the etheric body. Being aware of sexual energy and knowing how to work with and conduct it takes sex to the level of the sacred. Through meditation, visualization, and breath work, you will learn how to use erotic energy to infuse your life with magick and vitality.

Breath. Our society minimizes the importance of the conscious breath. Yet breathing is the foundation for life—and in sex, it is especially important. Breath guides your awareness, and because energy follows awareness (as sound healer and author Tom Kenyon so aptly put), breath guides energy. To move energy through your body when practicing sacred sex and sex magick, you use your breath and your will. Beyond that, breath helps you expand the possibilities of pleasure because holding your breath stops the flow of energy in your body. This can feel contradictory. I can say that committing to a breath work practice changed my life. It helped me find a sense of stability and peace in chaos, and it has helped me feel more deeply than I had before, especially during sex. Breath work is a fundamental practice for any spiritual tradition, and it makes sex more fun, powerful, present, and embodied, which leads to . . .

Embodiment. Embodiment is an umbrella term for practices that help you feel present in the physical self. Embodiment is a way of being in-body. Like breath work, it's not something we're taught in Western culture, which values the mind, brain, and logic more than it does intuition, inner guidance, and inner knowing—the latter of which only come from tuning into the body and honoring its truth. To live the path of sacred sexuality means living in the physical. *The mind may be the origin, but the body is where sacred sexuality lives.* There are many ways of experiencing and sustaining embodiment, and like sexuality itself, it will ebb and flow. Embodiment can be found through breath, movement (like yoga), conscious sex, masturbation, sound, dance, and affirmations, all of which will be woven through this book.

Glamour. Glamour isn't something you'll find as a tool of sacred sexuality in other sources, and that's because it's often not seen as very valuable. But it is a cornerstone of my own practice. Glamour is anything that conceals what lies beneath it, such as clothing, scent, makeup, and the like, so it can be considered a subset of embodiment. As any magician, occultist, or witch will tell you, there's an array of correspondences for colors, scents, and symbols, meaning an energetic or vibrational connection. (Roses are used for love magick, for example, because they are connected to Goddesses of Love and are also aphrodisiacs.) One way to amplify the power of a ritual—especially one as evocative and emotional as a sacred sex ritual—is by adorning yourself in corresponding colors, scents, symbols, and fabrics to align with your intention. Beyond this, glamour allows you to transform how you feel about yourself, which can be important in erotic rituals. Spirituality and magick transform you from the inside out, but glamour transforms you from the outside in. And when you combine these two practices, their power increases exponentially.

Movement. Movement is perhaps the most obvious of our tools, because sacred sex requires both physical and energetic movement. Movement is a path to embodiment because it helps you become spatially aware of the self and offers a way for you to circulate energy throughout your body. Movement of any kind can help, but dance, yoga, martial arts, and tai chi offer particularly beneficial results because they combine energetic awareness and physical movement. Dancing around your room, practicing yoga from YouTube, or just jumping up and down and shaking out your body all have the same effect. Being comfortable and aware of your body is a foundational aspect of sacred sex. Feeling the way your hips move, feeling how different movements can cause energy to react and respond, and allowing your body to lead and guide your awareness are all ways to weave the sensual into the mundane.

Masturbation. Last but not least is what I would consider one of the most important tools of sacred sexuality. Masturbation, or making self-love, is about connecting to your sexuality in a way that is pleasurable *for you*. There's a ton of shame and stigma around masturbation, even in this day and age, and one of the tenets of sacred sexuality is undoing these beliefs. Like low-stakes exposure therapy, one way to move against this ingrained belief around masturbation is to masturbate! Masturbation allows you access to what sex feels like for *you*. Not for your partner, not for the way your partner makes you feel, but *to and for you*. When you spend time in ritual masturbation, or exploring masturbation in a sacred space, you can begin to notice what pleasure is like in your body. You notice your desires and

---

A Note on Raising Energy

Throughout this book, you'll see the term *raising energy*. The definition takes two expressions. On one hand, during a spell or ritual, you will raise energy, or do something like masturbating or practicing sex magick, chanting, or dancing, to raise the state of being within yourself to a higher level of consciousness as a way of fueling your intention. You literally raise energy to charge a working, kind of like charging your phone to get it to full power. During sex magick specifically, you also raise energy up your spine, this time by using breath and awareness to literally guide sexual energy up your body, to again embolden or charge your working. I will guide you in which version of "raising energy" I mean for each ritual or meditation.

where the energy pools and shifts and expands. Then you have a foundation you can share with others, and for energy work, embodiment, and sex magick. If you have resistance or shame, take it slow. Begin by caressing yourself (like with a gentle hug or self-massage, for example), and add a bit more touch each time you return. No matter how much sex you're having with others, returning to your self in this way can balance your energetic equilibrium.

CREATING A SACRED
MASTURBATION PRACTICE

Masturbation is a form of sacred sex during which you get to decide your own pleasure. Through masturbation, you claim your autonomy by fulfilling your own needs. You are able to recognize what feels good in your body and what it feels like for erotic energy to course through you. You get to meet yourself sexually, so that when you share this with others, you're more able to communicate your wants.

One of the practices I invite you in to is creating a sacred self-love practice. This means ritualizing your self-pleasure routine:

- Before you begin masturbating, build your sacred space. Dim the lights or drape scarves over your lamps (carefully!) to diffuse the light. Light incense or candles. Play sexy music or ambient sounds. Be sure your phone is on silent and that you can have the time you need—even if it's five minutes—to be present.

- Cleanse any toys by running them through sacred smoke such as lavender, copal, or rose and banishing any negative or stuck energy, giving your body an energetic clean slate. Light the incense or herbs and blow out the flame so there's only a smolder left and then pass the toys through the smoke, visualizing anything that feels negative or stuck drifting away.

- Wear something—or nothing—that makes you feel beautiful, handsome, or sexy. Put on red lipstick, brush your hair, spritz on your favorite cologne, put on your favorite leather cuffs—do what you need to do to seduce yourself. Pay attention to your breath, allow it to expand your awareness, and see this as a bridge back into your body.

- Incorporate something outside of your usual reserves. If you usually watch porn, try reading erotica. If you usually read erotica, try listening to it or watching porn. Try something new.

- Keep a masturbation diary to help you unpack what works for you and what doesn't. You can be as detailed as you want (or not). You can write what you wore, what toys you used, if you watched porn or read erotica, how long you masturbated for, and if you had any orgasms (and if so, what it was like, how many you had, etc.). When you start practicing sex magick—or if you already do—you can include your intention and what other tools you used to complement it.

- Try new positions to change how pleasure feels in your body.

- Play with celibacy or committing to erotic exploration for a certain number of days. Take a break from masturbating to build up sexual energy—or masturbate every day for a certain number of days. Maybe you take five days off from masturbation, then masturbate every day for five days, and then start the cycle again. Get creative, and have fun.

- Incorporate other forms of touch. Use a feather to caress your skin, your nails to scratch, a flower to smell and press against your thighs and cheek. Give yourself a massage as foreplay. The point is to engage with touch in unexpected ways.

- See yourself as your own lover, and answer your own needs. Seeing yourself in relationship with your sexual self is transformative because you have the chance to ask, "What do I want right now?" and then give it to yourself. Instead of waiting for something or someone to come to the rescue, you can answer your own prayers.

Sexuality is about finding your edge, so if something feels like a huge *yuck*, sit with it and allow it to unfold, because it may be exactly what you need to explore. As always, you are the best judge of what makes sense, so come back to your own center as you decide what will serve you as you are, right here, right now.

HONORING YOUR BOUNDARIES AND NON-NEGOTIABLES

No is a sacred word. Through a declaration of a "no," you commit yourself to what feels right by rejecting what does not. Although moaning, screaming, or purring "yes" may have a sexier feel, each time you say no draws you closer to a full-body yes.

To walk the path of the sacred sex devotee means radical vulnerability and honesty when it comes to engaging with yourself as a sexual being. This takes commitment. There's a reason so many people numb themselves during sex. It's much easier not to do this Great Work and instead simply surrender to whatever your partner wants. But if you're reading this book, part of you that recognizes that sexual power leaks into every aspect of your life. The openness necessary to dance and fuck through the path of sacred sexuality means clearly and honestly engaging with your desires. This isn't something that happens in one day, nor is it an experience that's one and done. As sexuality is fluid and ever-evolving, so, too, do your desires change and develop and blossom and spiral. This means taking the time to check in with yourself and what you want as you begin engaging with new partners or new sexual experiences, and as you move more deeply on the path of the sacred slut, erotic artist, sexually liberated wo/man, or whatever else calls to you. This means taking the time to feel what brings you pleasure and to consciously recognize what doesn't. That's where your nos come in.

The word *no* isn't often celebrated. Many people take it as a personal attack. But the truth is that engaging with a no is a radical act of aligning with your truth. And there is nothing more powerful than being grounded in your truth. There will be people and experiences you change your mind about and decide to say no to, and some of the people may not like that. Know it's not personal. Someone who doesn't accept your boundaries is someone who benefited from you not having them, and that is not on you. One of the keys of sacred sexuality is honoring your boundaries, your non-negotiables, and your nos. They are what allow you to show up without fear because they create a safe container for your experience. Your no is a declaration that you don't want to do something. Your boundaries are the expression of what you feel comfortable with and your desires around engaging erotically. And your non-negotiables are the things you absolutely don't want to try or explore.

Note: if you have a partner who is trying to wrestle a boundary or no, and who won't take your boundary, no, or non-negotiable as an answer, that's a red flag. It's one thing to have a discussion with someone around an aversion; it's another thing to have someone make you question your decision or try to convince you they know what's best for you. *No one knows you as well as you.* Someone who's not honoring this probably doesn't have the right mindset or maturity to engage in sacred sex, and you should say goodbye.

Although nos, boundaries, and non-negotiables aren't quite as vital when you're engaging in a sacred sex relationship with only yourself, it is through personal exploration that you can begin to unravel what doesn't feel right. By showing up to sex with others aware of your nos, you can more easily, confidently, and safely engage with your yes and begin to unravel what that looks like. When you lay the foundation of honoring your boundaries and non-negotiables, you are stepping into your sexual power. This is liberation! This is sexual freedom! The more you honor what feels right for you, the more expressed and confident you will be in sharing it. And from here, magick is born.

One last note: your nos, boundaries, and non-negotiables aren't static. Just because you have a no or non-negotiable right now doesn't mean that will always be the truth. They most likely will change depending on your partner, your comfort level with yourself, and your sexual experiences. This is wonderful, delightful, and perfect. As you evolve in practice, so will they. Let's begin to figure out what your yeses and nos look like.

CREATING A
YES/NO/MAYBE LIST

In the world of kink, new initiates are urged to create a yes/no/maybe list. In one column or section of a page, write down the things you know you love, or you know you want to explore. In the next section, write down the things you are curious about. In the last section, write down whatever it is that's a hard limit, an absolute no. The reason this is so valuable—and the reason that creating and maintaining this list is an ongoing practice—is because when you write down your desires, you connect to them in a concrete way.

While a yes/no/maybe list typically involves kinks and fetishes, like bondage and anal sex, for example, I want you to make a yes/no/maybe list for all the experiences you have in your inventory. This could be kissing, tickling, eye contact, domination and submission, missionary, orgasm denial, holding hands, worship—whatever you feel strongly about should be placed here. Make this as much of a ritual as you'd like. Get dressed up in something that makes you feel sexy, put on a favorite playlist, light incense or candles, and put your phone on silent. Grab your journal or sex magick grimoire, and take a moment to ground and center yourself with a couple of deep breaths. Begin as you feel called, using the following for inspiration.

Yes: Write what you love to explore sexually and that which you know you want to try.

Maybe: Write what you're curious about, what you're open to exploring, and what makes you a bit nervous but in a good way.

No: Write what you know you don't want to try and what you recognize is a hard limit.

If you're not sure of what goes in each column, take this time to explore using the prompts below, noting what intrigues and interests you and what does not.

- Read books on kink or BDSM
- Read erotica
- Watch porn
- Journal around your favorite and least-favorite sexual experiences or about the sexual experiences you've seen in media, art, or porn that have lit your inner fire
- Pull tarot or oracle cards with the intention of erotic exploration
- Revisit old journals or diaries in which you've recounted sexual experiences or fantasies
- Spend time meditating on your sexuality, on your desires, and on what does and does not feel good in your body

Once you're done with your yes/no/maybe list, look over it. Remember to practice self-compassion, knowing that whatever's on this list is worthy of celebration, and that it will change and transform. Come back to it often, adding to it, changing it, or deleting things. This is a forever work in progress, one that reflects where you are in the present, and not something that defines your sexuality for the rest of time.

THE EMPRESS:
THE ARCHETYPE THAT OPENS THE DOOR
FOR EROTIC POTENTIAL

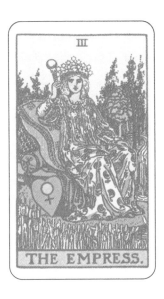

The third key in the tarot deck is the Empress, the Divine Mother sitting atop the throne of abundance, holding the scepter of power in her right hand, adorned by a crown of twelve stars—one for each of the zodiac signs—pregnant with the potential of all things, beside her the shield in the shape of a heart with the symbol for Venus carved into it. As the corresponding major arcana card for the planet and accompanying energy of Venus, the Empress represents pleasure, fertility, sensuality, creativity, sexuality, and love. She is an invitation into the senses, and even though the Empress is depicted as a woman, it doesn't mean her energy is gendered. To be alive in the world means having boundaries and a body, and this is what the feminine represents. The Empress is the way in which the energy of sexual, sensual expression; embodied love; and enjoyment can come to fruition. She acts as guardian and gateway to sacred sexuality because she *is* sacred sexuality.

It is the Empress who greets you as you step into your sexual power, inviting you to view pleasure as a sacrament, the body as a fertile playing ground for transcendence, and beauty as a vehicle for transporting you to other planes. The Empress is the Goddess of Love, inviting you to the world of Divine Erotic as a means of self-worship and cosmic consciousness.

The Empress raises all expressions of the heart by showing you how this in itself is a door to sacred sex. It can be about love, without being about being *in* love. To connect to the Empress as an erotic archetype means tapping into the creative, intuitive, and expansive wisdom of the Divine Feminine. It means recognizing your emotional nature as an esoteric path to your sexuality. This means seeing your feelings as fertile soil for your desires and wishes, a doorway to ecstasy, gnosis, and evolution. The Empress reflects the feminine unfiltered by patriarchy, rooted in the transcendent power of the heart, love, and the earth. The Empress is knowledge grounded in the body, in the connection of the self to all that is.

The Empress is the form and body, and her counterpart, the Emperor, acts as the igniting force or power. Alchemically, the Empress is salt, the body, while the Emperor is sulfur, which is what energizes the salt. While the Empress invites you into your sexuality, the Emperor invites you into your power and asks you to use it wisely. This means not wielding your sexuality to hurt, manipulate, or harm, but using it to bring yourself into a state of higher evolution, and by doing so, inviting others to do the same. Correspondent to the cardinal fire sign of Aries—the first sign of the zodiac that initiates spring on the spring equinox—the Emperor is the flame that lights the candle of the Empress. Together, they are initiators in the Divine Erotic.

The Empress says to revel in the body, the skin, the sensual.
To surrender to pleasure, to ecstasy, the sexual.
The Emperor says to remember your power, your strength,
your roots. To own your desires, your body, your fuel.
The Empress is the door to the sacred sexual, and
the Emperor is the window in which you can gaze
through at your fullest potential.

Preparing for Ritual:
Setting Up the Space, Grounding, and Shielding

Before you begin any ritual, it's imperative that you have your psyche, space, and spirit all set and aligned. This means ensuring the mundane world is conducive to your spiritual exploits and that your spiritual self is protected and grounded to the earth. *I will be referring to these opening steps for ritual throughout this book, so make sure you're familiar with them.*

SETTING UP THE SPACE. Before you begin your spell or ritual, get yourself in order. Light some candles and incense, gather your supplies, and make sure you won't be disturbed for the duration of the working. Take care of any pets, ensure any roommates or partners know not to disturb you (even if this means leaving a sign on your door), and put your phone on silent. Dim the lights, put on some solfeggio frequencies or ambient music if you wish, and change into something that makes you feel like a sexpot. Clean and tidy your space, and make sure you have a perimeter of at least three feet to work in. Then, take care of yourself! You may want to avoid eating for an hour or two before your ritual if your body allows. You don't want to be full, and you also don't want to be so hungry it's all you can think about. Find a middle ground for yourself. Make sure you feel present in the flesh and sexy as fuck. You are the most important part of any ritual, darling, so treat yourself as the main character, and adorn yourself accordingly.

GROUNDING AND SHIELDING. Once your space is set, you will want to get your etheric, astral, and physical body ready for the working ahead. You do this through grounding, connecting to the earth below you and the heavens above you, so you can draw energy from that terrestrial and celestial energy instead of from yourself or others. That way you're not creating any sort of energetic deficit on this plane, but instead pulling from the infinite and limitless.

Find a comfortable seat, either sitting up or lying down with your spine straight. Come back to your breath, allowing it to guide you into the present moment. As you feel centered, find a comfortable rhythm of breath as you feel your belly fill with air as you inhale and feel it deflate as you exhale. Do this a few times. Begin to visualize the base of your spine turning into roots or a golden cord that reaches out and digs into the ground, all the way into the crystal core of the earth. These roots or cord are fed golden, healing light that moves back up your spine, through your entire body, out the crown of your head, and all the way into the heavens. White healing light from above then pours through the crown of your head, moving down through every inch of your body, meeting the terrestrial energy from below at your heart center. Feel the energies of the terrestrial and celestial realms meeting and swirling at your heart space and then breathe into this like you're expanding a bubble. This bubble extends from your heart and grows and pushes out any negative energy from your being and space as it does. Eventually, this protective sphere or circle of light contains your whole body—and several feet above, below, and to each side of you—enclosing your ritual space in its protective energy. Only that which vibrates in 100 percent Divine light and aligns with highest good can move through this protective sphere. If you are doing this with a partner or partners, each person should perform this exercise and then you can visualize each of your spheres of protection combining to form a giant sphere that encompasses you all.

I will be referring to this method of grounding and protecting throughout this book and will call it "grounding and shielding" as shorthand in the beginning steps of a ritual.

CLOSING AND GROUNDING. After a ritual, it's important that you finish and then close the grounding. To do this, you perform the exercises again but in the opposite way. As you're ready to close the ritual, find a comfortable position. Feel the roots or golden cord moving from the base of your spine into the earth once again and then visualize them moving back into your body, where they dissolve into white light. Feel the connection with the cosmos above, moving this energy up your body and spine, through the crown of your head, and back into the heavens, where you allow it to dissolve. Then, feel the sphere of protection around you. With each breath, feel this sphere shrink and move back into your heart center, where it dissolves and reenters your energy field. You may press your forehead and then the crown of your head into the floor, like in child's pose, and release any excess energy back into the earth, where it will be reabsorbed.

I will be referring to this practice of ending a ritual as "closing and grounding" throughout this book.

CREATING AN ALTAR
FOR YOUR SACRED SEXUALITY

Because sexuality is an ephemeral force—meaning it's something you *feel* and don't necessarily *see*—it can be helpful to have visual reminders of your connection to your erotic power. One way of doing this is by creating an altar, or an energetic and magickal focal point of a space. This is where you can leave offerings to deities you work with, lay out tarot cards, pray, and connect with and come back to your sexual essence. Because this book is rooted in magick, and because I am a lifelong devotee to both the Goddess and witchcraft, there are plenty of magickal elements woven in, including altar work.

Sex usually happens in the bedroom, so I suggest making your altar there. This way, you begin the process of shifting your bedroom from a mundane space to a sacred one. By bringing awareness and intention into your bedroom, and by erecting and establishing an altar here, you are inviting in a sense of reverence, a space in which your relationship to the Divine Erotic can take root and grow.

When you're creating an altar, it's important to remember that this is a physical reflection of the most sacred altar you will ever have: *you*. You are a living, breathing erotic temple where the cosmos manifest through flesh and pleasure. A physical altar acts as a reminder and reflection of the power within you, of the loving magick you connect with when you walk the spiral path of sacred sex. Plus, when you begin to practice sex magick, it can act as an energetic home for your magickal workings.

CREATING AN ALTAR

Step 1: Decide where to put your altar

Before you get to creating your altar, you'll want to figure out where to put it. I have an altar on top of my dresser, although you could place yours on your nightstand, bookshelf, desk, vanity, or counter. Again, because the intention of this altar is to connect with your sexuality, put it somewhere in your bedroom (or if you have a sex dungeon, that works, too!), although you of course may place it somewhere else. If you don't feel comfortable having a permanent altar or simply can't, you can keep your supplies in a box that you take out and set up whenever you need it. Once you have decided on your space, you may wish to clean it and wipe it down with rose water, Florida water, or Moon water.

Step 2: Gather your supplies

With your space set, next collect your supplies. One of the things to keep in mind is beauty and picking objects for your altar that have harmony and resonance to make your space more powerful and appealing. Think of items that relate to your sexuality: things you've inherited (like lace or jewelry) or bought or created (like tarot cards, sex toys, or art). Consider erotic art, candles (especially red and pink because these are colors of sex and love, respectively, or green, the color of Venus), tarot or oracle cards, sex toys, condoms, lube, jewelry, lingerie, crystals, books of erotica or love poetry, letters, perfume, makeup like lipstick, flowers, and whatever else helps feed your erotic inspiration. When you leave things on your altar, you are also imbuing them with sacred energy.

Step 3: Arrange your altar

Once you have your objects chosen, arrange them on your altar. You may center an object like a piece of art or a favorite book and then add other items like candles, sex toys, tarot and oracle cards, and crystals. The point is to make a space that is both exciting and beautiful to look at. Every time you gaze at your altar, you should be reminded of your commitment to your sexuality and to the practice of honoring this as sacred. Your altar can be as PG-13 or NC-17 as you wish. It doesn't matter. What matters is how *you* feel about it and that it brings you joy.

Step 4: Cleanse and bless

Once you have arranged your altar, cleanse it with water (like spring water, rose water, Florida water, or oil or perfume) and consecrate it with sacred smoke (like frankincense, myrrh, rose, cedar, ethically sourced palo santo, or incense). This clears your altar and its objects of any stagnant energy or energy that doesn't belong to you and infuses it with your intention of creating a portal to the Divine Erotic. You can use the following cleansing and consecrating practice or make your own. Honor whatever resonates with your own practice, tradition, or lineage.

Sprinkle water in each corner of your altar, and say the following:

I cleanse this altar in the name of my sacred sexuality, fluid and creative, inspiring and evolving. I release and banish all energies stopping me from standing firmly in my truth and most Divine Erotic capability. And so it is.

Then, lighting your herbs, incense, or resin, pass the smoke through your altar, moving counterclockwise first to banish stagnant energy and then clockwise to draw in positive energy, saying the following:

I consecrate this altar in the name of my sacred sexuality, fiery and passionate, expressive and ecstatic. I erect this altar through my own erotic power. Only that which honors my True Will and works in my highest favor is welcome. This or something better for the highest good of all involved, and so it is.

After, take some time to close your eyes and feel the space you've created for yourself. You may meditate, pray, or hold your palms above your altar, feeling cosmic energy moving through your body and out your hands. Stay here as long as you need, reveling in what you've manifested.

CONSECRATING A SACRED SEX GRIMOIRE

Magick is a creative act, but it also requires a scientific approach. To enact the most potent magick possible, you need to be able to see what's worked, and what hasn't, so you can be intentional in what to take with you on your journey. The easiest way to begin doing this is by keeping a magickal diary or record, known as a grimoire. A grimoire is a journal of all your magickal workings, musings, inspiration, and ideas. Your grimoire will be customized to your interests, to what sort of journal-keeping suits you best, and to whatever it is that influences your practice. Although many witches choose to have one grimoire for all their magick, I find that keeping separate ones for different parts of my practice is extremely helpful. Not only is it much easier to go back and reflect this way, it also feels extra potent, special, and honestly *sexy* to have a grimoire all for my most subversive and sexual magick. As always, what's important is that you start where you are.

What separates a journal from a grimoire is the act of consecration, which means imbuing the journal itself with intention and energy, specifically by using the element of fire. In the following pages, find a guide for consecrating your Sacred Sex Grimoire. Adapt it as you wish.

Try to perform this ritual during a full Moon
(the peak of Lady Luna's energy),
although it can be done at any time.

What you need: Your grimoire, herbs or resins and a fireproof dish, a lighter, coal if you're using a resin, a chalice or cup of water (Moon water, rose water, Florida water, holy water, spring or tap water, etc.), and any sex toys and lube you want to use.

Step 1: Pick out your Sacred Sex Grimoire

It's said that investing in your magickal supplies acts as an offering, devotion, and amplification of your intention. If you have the means to invest a little and feel called to do so, go for it. But know that by no means is this necessary, and the Notes app on your iPad or a $2 composition book from the drugstore can be just as powerful to work with as a $50 leather-bound journal. I like to use the same Leuchtturm1917 Composition size notebooks for all my grimoires, and I buy different colors depending on what I use it for. My Sacred Sex

Grimoire is magenta pink and holds the energy of my relationship with the Divine Erotic beautifully.

When you pick out your grimoire, *some things to think about are*: Do you want this to be digital or handwritten? Is the notebook or program you're using easy to write in? If you're doing this digitally, is this file something safe and something you can back up? Is the journal weighty enough to be substantial but light enough that you can bring it with you? Once you've figured out your journal, you'll be able to consecrate it.

Step 2: Set up your space, ground, and shield

Now is the time to set up your space, ground, and shield, as laid out earlier in this chapter.

Step 3: Cleanse with water

Now that you're ready to consecrate your grimoire, begin by cleansing it using water. Take a moment to hold your palms over your chalice or cup, connecting to the energies from above and below you once again. Feel this move through your palms and into the water, imbuing it with the energy of the Divine Erotic. When you feel the water is charged, dip your fingers into it and press them onto your grimoire. (You can also sprinkle the water very lightly, ensuring you don't drip enough to damage anything if you have an electronic grimoire.)

Say the following, or rewrite it to suit your needs:

Through the cleansing powers of water
I consecrate this grimoire with my desires.
I align this grimoire with the Divine Erotic,
Releasing anything negative, heavy, and toxic.
May any energies not of me be banished from herein completely.

On all planes and all ways this grimoire is cleansed,
For the use of Sacred Sex, magick, and my sensual depths.

You may wish to take a moment and hold your palms over your grimoire as you feel waves of cleansing energy moving through it, sweeping away any energy it may have picked up in the process of getting to you.

Step 4: Consecrate with sacred smoke

Repeat this same process, but with sacred smoke, which holds the vibration of elemental fire and air. You may repeat the visualization with your herbs or resin, holding your palms above and feeling the energies from above and below moving through you and imbuing your herbs or resin with the vibration of the Divine Erotic. If you are using sacred herbs (lavender, mugwort, and ethically sourced palo santo are all good choices), light them and then blow them out so they smolder. If you are using resin, light the activated charcoal piece, wait until it sparks all the way through and is red or white, and then place the resin on top. Once you have some smoke going, pass your grimoire through it, visualizing the smoke imbuing it with the energy of sacred sex. As you do this, say the following, rewriting or adapting as you see fit:

By the power of the sacred flame
Brought forth from the highest, and through every plane
I consecrate this Sacred Sex Grimoire
To serve my growth, my magick, and my Divinely Erotic soul.
May this fire and smoke imbue this grimoire
With everything I need to grow and evolve,
In alignment with my highest sexual self.

This grimoire is consecrated and magically prepared.
So mote it be.

Take a moment and hold your palms over your grimoire as you feel the passion of fire and sexual energy moving through it, charging it with your intention, and transforming it into a sacred container of your magick.

Step 5 (optional): Sex magick and anoint with sexual fluids
So now comes the option for some sex magick. Begin to masturbate. Allow yourself to be totally present and feel the energy you're raising coursing through your body. As you get closer and closer to orgasm, or as close as possible, take your Sacred Sex Grimoire in your hands and pour all this energy into it through your palms, staying here until you feel all the energy moved into it. Then, in the afterglow, hold the vision of this grimoire being a sacred container for your explorations with the Divine Erotic. Once you feel done, take some sexual fluid and anoint your grimoire with a small bit of it (somewhere that won't leave a mark) as you say the following, writing or adapting it as you see fit:

With the sexual energy from my own body,
I consecrate this Sacred Sex Grimoire, purely and erotically.
May this be a vessel for my explorations of sex and spirit,
And inspire me in all ways so I may grow with it.
This or something better for the highest good of all involved,
This Sacred Sex Grimoire is consecrated, and the working is done.
So it is, and so mote it be!

Take a second to hold your grimoire in any way that resonates: place your palms on it, or hold it against your heart. Send it all the energy within you, all the energy you've raised and connected with. Know that this grimoire is an ally, a support system, and a sacred mirror. Continue connecting with it as long as you'd like.

Step 6: Close and ground
When you're ready to close the ritual, find a comfortable position and then perform the closing and grounding exercises.

You officially have a consecrated Sacred Sex Grimoire! You may wish to record your experience from this ritual within it or write a blessing for your journey. Include the sign the Sun and Moon are in, the date, and any other pertinent information. And so it is.

JOURNAL QUESTIONS

Although journaling may not seem like the most impactful way to connect with your sexual self, my hope is that after trying it, you think otherwise. Like anything else, journaling is what you make of it, and creating an inspiring environment—and wearing something that helps you feel into yourself as a sensual being—is not only recommended but encouraged as you answer the journal questions in each chapter. It is also a really good way to get to know yourself erotically because you don't have to pretend to be anything you're not. It is a completely safe and private environment where you can be as real, raw, explicit, dramatic, over the top, and sensual as you want.

Answer whichever of the following questions resonate with you, and use them to go off on whatever tangents feel right. Create a mind map, doodle, free write—or not. It's up to you. The point is to inspire you to dig deeper. Allow the questions to be a jumping-off point, and if you wish, you can answer them in your Sacred Sex Grimoire.

I always recommend turning journaling into a ritual of its own by setting up a sacred space. Light incense or candles or diffuse oil, slip into something silky or perhaps some lace or leather, and put on your sexy playlist or ambient noise like a crackling fireplace. Pull oracle or tarot cards if it's in your practice, and gather any supportive energies like pets or crystals. Take a moment to breathe, center yourself or meditate, and then, as you feel ready, answer. Once again, this preparatory ritual for journaling will be the same throughout this book.

- How do I define sacred sexuality? Sacred sex?
- What are my goals and intentions that I hope to get out of this book?
- How has my relationship with my sexuality and sex begun to evolve and shift since the beginning of this book, if at all?
- How can I begin to make my relationship with my erotic essence more conscious and intentional? What sort of simple rituals can I work with?
- What in my life brings me pleasure? How can I tap into this more frequently, to bring more pleasure into other areas of my life?
- What traditions of sacred sex am I most familiar with and inspired by? How does this show up in my own cultures, spiritual practice, or tradition?

- How did creating a yes/no/maybe list help me intensify my understanding of my desires? What surprised me? What did I learn?
- What shame, fear, and guilt am I still releasing? What practices, rituals, and affirmations can I work with to more easily let go of these outdated beliefs?
- How does honoring my nos, boundaries, and non-negotiables help me stand more firmly in my power? How can I practice honoring these in my day-to-day life?
- What do the Tower and Star cards mean to me? How can they help me in releasing and rewriting my beliefs around sex?
- What do the Empress and the Emperor cards mean to me? How can they act as erotic archetypes that guide me in this journey?

A TAROT SPREAD FOR UNDERSTANDING YOUR RELATIONSHIP TO SACRED SEX

Alongside the journal questions at the end of each chapter, I also will be including a tarot spread to help you unravel these themes in a more symbolic way. You can also use an oracle deck, which is created by artists and don't conform to a single structure as the tarot does. The tarot spread in this chapter is meant to act as a mirror to the Divine Erotic. There are no wrong cards and no wrong interpretation—there only is what comes up. Use the following to help gain perspective on your journey, and remember to have plenty of self-compassion along the way.

Working with Tarot

Before you begin pulling cards, you may wish to turn this into a ritual. The steps for preparing your space for a reading will be the same throughout this book. Wear something that makes you feel sensual, and set the mood by lighting candles or incense. You may meditate or practice breath work as you formulate the question you'll be asking the cards, which can be specific or general, such as, "What is my current relationship to sacred sex?" Take the time to shuffle the cards as you ask your question, stopping when you feel ready. You may cut the deck by dividing it into two or three piles and then putting one of the piles on the top. When you feel called, pull your cards and record your interpretations in your Sacred Sex Grimoire. And so it is.

Card 1: What is my current relationship with sacred sexuality?

Card 2: How I can harness this as a path of magick?

Card 3: What beliefs should I release and let go of?

Card 4: What supportive erotic beliefs can I invite in instead?

Card 5: What message does this card give me for my journey?

AFFIRMATIONS

We'll also work with affirmations throughout this book. Affirmations help you develop more optimistic and positive ways of seeing yourself, and in this case, to develop a more meaningful relationship with your sexuality. Affirmations are here to help you dissolve the binary of sacred and profane so you can see your eroticism as another aspect of your spiritual self.

Working with Affirmations

Throughout this book, you will be invited to work with affirmations. There are many ways to do this. My suggestion is to do them while you gaze at the reflection of your nondominant eye in the mirror. (If you're left-handed, your nondominant eye is your right eye; if you're right-handed, it's your left eye.) Speak your affirmations out loud three times before moving on to the next one, and repeat every day if you can. The more often you say them, the better. You can even schedule an alarm so you don't forget. You can also write them on a sticky note or piece of paper and tape them to your mirror, record them in your Sacred Sex Grimoire, or turn them into a graphic and use them as your phone wallpaper.

If you've never worked with affirmations, it's normal to feel silly or embarrassed as you start. Just remember to be compassionate with yourself and remind yourself that you're doing this so you can grow and become more centered. The more you do it, the less weird it will feel.

- I walk the path of sacred sex.
- I dance the dance of the Divine Erotic.
- I am both sacred and profane.
- I am both spiritual and sexual.
- I claim my sexual power.
- I own my sexual sovereignty.
- I am rooted in my erotic independence.
- I love sex and claim the title of someone who loves sex with pride.
- I release all outdated beliefs around my sexuality with ease.
- I reclaim my sexuality as my own and as a path to sacred embodiment.
- I am a sex God/dess, and I work with my sexuality as a path to empowerment.
- I am a Priest/ess of my own pleasure on the path of sacred sex.
- My sexuality is my own and belongs to no one but me.
- I share my sexuality with those I see fit, without shame or guilt.

A TALISMAN AND AMULET SPELL WITH THE TOWER AND THE STAR TO RELEASE SHAME AND CALL IN SEXUAL SOVEREIGNTY

In this ritual, you will set up the foundation for your practice with sacred sexuality by casting a spell—or a magickal working that uses action, energy, and intention to manifest your desire—to release shame and draw in sexual freedom, sovereignty, and liberation. You will be creating an amulet to keep shame away and a talisman to draw sexual sovereignty in and then charging them both with sexual energy so they manifest on the material plane. Welcome to the world of sex magick.

What you need: A few pieces of paper, a journal or grimoire, a pen and pencil, the Tower and Star tarot cards if you have them, and scissors.

Optional: A black chime candle, a white chime candle, candleholders, a lighter or matches, sex toys, and lube.

You may practice this ritual during a new Moon or a full Moon. Since you will be banishing and calling in at the same time, either of these phases will work.

Read over the ritual before you begin it to get familiar with it, and to plan and adapt accordingly.

Step 1: Set up the space, ground, and shield

Now it's time to begin the ritual! Set up the space and ground and shield as laid out earlier in this chapter. You can also invite in the elements or perform the Lesser Banishing Ritual of the Pentagram (LBRP) or the Hexagram (LBRH) or whatever other rituals you'd like. Take the time to call upon any deities or guides you work with in terms of sexuality, erotic expression, and embracing the transgressive. If you don't know what I'm talking about, don't worry—you can still call upon the cosmos, the Divine, your higher self, or your higher sexual self. Use whatever words feel right for you, trusting in your expression and in your heart. You can use the following as framework:

> *I call upon my higher sexual self, my most sensual self, my erotic truth, to guide me in this ritual of releasing shame and reclaiming my sexual sovereignty. May I be held, protected, and led by the universe so I can stand firmly in my power, as I am meant to. And so it is.*

Once you've called in this energy, evoked, or invoked, take a moment to breathe and feel it. Allow the presence of your higher self to make itself known. Even if you don't feel or sense anything, trust in the magick. Know it's working.

Step 2: Connect with the Tower and Star cards

You will be constructing an amulet, which keeps something away, using the Tower card to release sexual shame, guilt, or whatever is holding you back from owning your erotic truth. Then you will be constructing a talisman, which draws something toward you, using the Star card to call in sexual autonomy, confidence, and power.

Take a moment to meditate on each of these cards, referring to pages 21–22 for background on what they mean. Ask yourself how the Tower represents what you want to let go of, what thoughts and beliefs you need to strip power from. Then write a sentence to embody your intention for releasing this, using the present or past tense as you do so. An example: *I release shame, guilt, and fear around expressing myself sexually, around my self-expression, around standing fully in my erotic power.*

Then do the same for the Star, but this time concentrate on what you want to bring into your practice of sacred sex, and which beliefs, feelings, thoughts, and experiences will support this journey. An example: *I draw in strength, power, and confidence around my sexuality and desires. I am grounded in my erotic power, and my life is a ritual of sensuality.*

If you work with Hermetic Qabalah, you may wish to connect with the paths of these cards, looking at the gates and the Divine names, archangels, angelic choirs, and mundane chakras they connect to. You can also look at their corresponded Hebrew letter for more depth, or scry into the cards to understand how they relate to your erotic essence.

Step 3: Make the amulet and talisman

Construct your amulet and talisman. There are a few options (and see the section on sigil magick on page 110 for more details):

- Form a sigil, or a charged symbol, using the intentions you created in the last step. Write out your intention on a piece of paper, and cross out all the repeating letters. You may also cross out the vowels so you're only left with consonants. Then, using a pencil, combine and layer the remaining letters on top of one another to create a symbol. *Do this for the Tower/amulet and what you want to release and then repeat for the Star/talisman and what you want to draw in.* You will have two separate sigils. When you are satisfied with the shapes, draw each with a black or red pen on a clean piece of paper, and draw a circle around them.

- Pick a word or a couple of words to represent your intention for the amulet (what you want to banish) and then a word or couple of words to represent your intention with the talisman (or what you want to draw in). Use a witch's sigil wheel, which has all the letters of the alphabet in a circle, by tracing from letter to letter for each word. When you're done, use a black or red pen to draw the resulting sigil for the amulet on a piece of paper and the sigil for the talisman on another piece of paper. You will have two separate sigils to work with.

- You may also use your intention to channel or free draw a symbol for an amulet inspired by the Tower and a symbol for the talisman inspired by the Star.

No matter what you do, cut out the two pieces of paper, *making sure to remember which is which by writing "Tower/amulet" on the back of the one correlated to them and "Star/talisman" on the back of the other.*

Step 4 (optional): Anoint and light the candles

If you want to work with candle magick, anoint your black candle with protective oil, banishing oil, olive oil, or something like dragon's blood, spreading it over the candle from wick to base, or from the middle of the candle to each end. Add herbs like bay leaves, frankincense, or mugwort on the candle in the same way, sprinkling just a bit on it, or placing the herbs on a piece of paper and rolling the candle in them. Then place the Tower card on your altar with your anointed black candle on top or beside.

Black banishes and white attracts, so now anoint your white candle to draw in. Use honey, olive oil, or manifesting oil, either spreading it from the base of the candle to the top or from each end to the middle. Add herbs like rose, cinnamon, chamomile, or jasmine in the same way, sprinkling just a bit on the candle, or placing the herbs on a piece of paper and rolling the candle in them. Then place the Star card on the right of the Tower card on your altar, with your anointed white candle on top or beside.

Take a moment to reconnect with your intention, with your higher sexual self, or whatever deities, beings, or energies you called in before. Feel your power. If it's in your practice to intone the Divine names, archangels, angelic choirs, and mundane chakras of certain spheres on the Tree of Life to support your work, you may do so at this time, either before or after lighting the candle.

As you feel ready, light the candle and know that you are drawing in power from the cosmos, from the unmanifest, helping it descend into this world to carry out your will and desire. Gaze at the flame, and read out loud your intentions, starting with what you want to release and moving to what you're calling in. You may wish to close with "This or something better for the highest good of all involved, in alignment with my True Will."

Step 5: Charge the amulet and talisman

If you are not working with candle magick, place the Tower card on your altar and then set the Star card to the right of it. Feel your power, and reconnect to your sacred essence. Read your intentions out loud, starting with what you are releasing and moving toward what you're calling in. You may wish to close your intentions with "This or something better for the highest good of all involved, in alignment with my will." Stay here as long as you like, journaling if it calls to you.

Now you will perform sex magick to charge the talismans. Gather whatever you need—lube, sex toys—and place your amulet and talisman within eyesight. Begin to masturbate as you focus on being engaged with your sexual power. Imagine how it will feel to be your most sexually sovereign and liberated self. Give yourself pleasure, and allow it to be an enriching experience, as you raise the sexual energy more and more, as you breathe into your erotic power. As you feel yourself get to the peak—aka orgasm, or as close as you can get—open your eyes, look at your talisman and amulet, and send the energy through your body, through the crown of your head, and into these objects. As you stay in the afterglow, you may place your talisman and amulet on your chest, visualizing your intention of being fully in your sexual power, without shame. Stay here as long as you'd like.

When you're done, place your amulet on top of the Tower card (under or beside the candle) and your talisman on top of the Star card (under or beside the candle).

If you don't want to charge this spell through sex magick, you can dance, move, chant, or do something else to physically raise energy. Then follow the process of sending energy into the amulet and talisman.

Step 6: Close the ritual

When you're ready to close the ritual, return to whatever position you began in. Come back to your breath. If you invited in any deities or guides, thank and dismiss them. If you invited in your higher sexual self, thank it using whatever words feel right, or adapt the following:

Higher, sensual self, grounded in my erotic truth, I thank you for joining me in this ritual of releasing shame and reclaiming my sexual sovereignty. Thank you for holding me, protecting me, and allowing me to be led by the universe. I stand firmly in my power. The ritual is closed, and you are dismissed. Thank you, thank you, thank you. So mote it be.

Now, perform the closing and grounding exercises. Thank yourself for this ritual of self-devotion as you feel the energy leaving.

Place your talisman and amulet in the back of your Sacred Sex Grimoire or keep them on your altar, in your sex toy drawer, or wherever you keep things like lingerie. Or feel free to burn them.

When you're done, connect with yourself and journal about your experience. Then eat some food, drink some water, and come back into your body. A postritual bath can really hit the spot.

If you lit candles, allow them to burn all the way down. (You can leave them in a sink.) If you can't let them burn down safely, snuff or fan them out—don't blow them out because this is said to blow out the magick—and then relight them the next time you reconnect to your intentions. If there's excess wax, throw it out in a garbage can at an intersection—the modern witch's crossroads—which disperses the spell's energy.

And so it is.

CHAPTER 2

Expanding Pleasure: Sex Ed 101

L et's get back to basics. Like the basic basics. Sex education? Doesn't that kind of take the *sexy* out of the whole thing? We have to start here, because there's a high likelihood that if you grew up in the United States, the sexual education you received in school was anything but comprehensive. And that's if you received any sexual education at all. As of 2021, only thirty states mandate both sex education and human immunodeficiency virus (HIV) education, and only eighteen states mandate that the lessons be medically accurate. Take into account that the sex education those states teach may be abstinence-based, and that there's more than likely no talk of pleasure, and you have a recipe for disaster.

True sex ed is vital for the sex mystic because it means taking an active interest in your sexuality. It means understanding your body and dispelling the myths that are ever so prevalent in ecstasy-crushing patriarchal cultures, whose view of pleasure is often centered on a man with a penis.

COMMON MYTHS
ABOUT SEX AND SEXUALITY

We won't be getting into the weeds here, but I do want to take time to dispel some of the most pervasive myths about sex you've probably heard, especially those of you with vulvas. And let's start there, because you might not know the difference between a vulva or vagina, or even what these are! The vagina is the birth canal; the vulva is the whole delectable package, including the exterior features, the clitoris, the labia majora and labia minora (the inner and outer lips), the urethral opening (where you pee), and the vaginal opening.

Because most sex studies have been done on those with penises, and more specifically men with penises, the norm for sexuality is likewise skewed. And vulvas or pussies and penises or dicks are made of the same stuff, as Emily Nagoski so refreshingly explains, but just arranged differently. This means that bodies behave and react in different ways. To be able to have the explosive sex life you want, you need to know what you're working with, and part of knowing what you're working with means throwing out old beliefs and patterns that society has taught you. Here are the main myths stopping you from living your best sex life. While this is in no way definite, my hope is that unpacking them begins your sex-positive sex ed journey.

MYTH I: VIRGINITY IS REAL, AND SEX = P + V

One of the most ingrained narratives in Western culture is that sex is the act of inserting a penis into a vagina, and that the first time this happens you "lose" something. Even more, losing your virginity is something to be celebrated for those with penises but for people with vulvas, girls, and women, it's shameful and inappropriate. This double standard infuses much of the way society speaks of sex.

I define sex as "anything with the potential to bring you an expansive sense of pleasure, with the possibility of orgasm." This can be masturbation or intercourse, or getting spanked or sitting in the sun naked. Sex is extremely personal, and your definition of it will reflect this. (Later in this chapter, you will be guided in writing your own definitions of sex, love, pleasure, and so on.) It's this binary, penis-in-vagina thinking that stops so many from having the sex life of their dreams. Seeing only one act as "real" sex creates a hierarchy in which anything else is not as intimate or important. That's BS.

The idea of virginity stems from this myth as well. In the ancient past, virginity was associated with belonging to oneself, reflected by the Virgin Goddesses like Artemis, Vesta, Isis, and Inanna, who were not defined by partners (and who were mostly unwed, except Isis) and were not sexually chaste. The modern puritanical idea of virginity has to do with the belief that the hymen, a fold of mucous membrane that partially encloses the vaginal opening, is broken the first time you have sex, which represents loss. The thing is, the hymen doesn't break. If a hymen tears or bruises, it heals like any other part of the body. And while the narrative of bleeding and experiencing some pain the first time you have penetrative sex is normal, the bleeding is more likely due to a vaginal tear and lack of lubrication than from tearing your hymen. Y'all, virginity is a social construct.

MYTH 2: PEOPLE WITH A PENIS CAN ONLY COME ONCE, AND COMING = EJACULATION

Did you know that people with penises can have internal orgasms? That means that if you have a penis, you can come without ejaculation, and if you're trained in the art of loving in this way, you can maintain an erection while you do so, sending the erotic energy and sperm back into your body. This form of sacred sexuality is known as ejaculation control or semen retention and is a tool used by tantrikas, sexual magicians, and others who practice sacred sex. Ejaculation control, or the process of stopping ejaculation to elongate the ritual of sex, is a method of sex magick that can make the person with the penis multiorgasmic—fun and functional if you're aiming for a magickal or mystical purpose. Ejaculation control can be done manually by placing the pointer, middle, and ring fingers around the base of the penis, pressing into the perineum, and applying pressure when you feel like you're about to come. Or you can sit in half lotus pose, with one leg straight out in front of you and one heel drawn as far back as possible under the buttocks, specifically under the perineum. You won't ejaculate with either of these methods, and you will lose your erection—but you can still have sex without a hard dick, so worry not.

For readers who are serious about their sacred sex studies, you can research other methods that will allow you to delay ejaculation while maintaining an erection. By using breath and energetic locks (where you contract muscles alongside breath work), known as bandhas in yogic tradition, you can circulate the sexual energy and semen from the penis back through the body. By lifting the pelvic floor, tightening the anus and perineum, and using the breath to guide this energy back into the body, internal orgasm and multiple orgasms are possible.

The key is practice. Practice as you masturbate, working with the three-finger lock, half lotus, and breath and locks to begin getting comfortable with changing your relationship with ejaculation. Figure out the sexual peak and limit of no return—the point where you feel like you're going to come and are unable to stop. If you practice with lovers, keep in mind some of the signs of "no return" are important. The testicles begin to pull into the body, a change in breath occurs, and precum (liquid that is ejaculated before semen, the body's form of a natural lubricant) may be ejaculated. By communicating with your partner, slowing down, deepening the breath, and practicing the root lock, you'll be on your way to coming without the cum in no time.

MYTH 3: THE CLIT IS SMALL AND UNIMPORTANT

Did you know that the clitoris is the only part of the human anatomy solely designed for pleasure? Did you know that it has more nerve endings than any other part of the body? Did you know it has legs? If you answered yes to any of these, congratulations! And if you said "No, what the actual fuck?" then, welcome, you are in the right place. Because the anatomy of those with vulvas is often ignored in scientific studies, it wasn't even until 1998 that Helen O'Connell discovered that there was such a thing as an internal clitoris.

The clitoris is the home of sensation. The nub, or visible part of the clitoris, which lies beneath the pubic mound, is what most people associate with this aspect of anatomy, although this is just the tip of the iceberg. The clitoris has two internal legs that extend from the nub of the clitoris on either side, encircling the vagina. The clitoris is to the vulva what the glans (or head) is to the penis. In total, the clitoris is composed of eighteen different parts, making it comparable to the genital structure of the penis. The penis and vulva have almost the same anatomy; it's just arranged differently and requires different forms of touch to reach their fullest potential.

If you have a vulva, or love someone with a vulva, or just want to be the most educated sex mystic or sex witch possible, this is key: pleasure should be democratic. As sex educator and author of the *Boudoir Bible* Betony Vernon states, "Understanding your body and that of your lovers allows you to create a map that will guide you both on your journeys to heightened sexual satisfaction."

MYTH 4: WETNESS = HORNINESS = AROUSAL = READINESS

Your body is an animal. And sometimes animals don't follow the rules. So is this true of the sexual being inside you. Namely, if you have a vulva or love and/or fuck someone with a vulva, this is true of the vaginal lubrication or wetness that may or may not happen when things begin to get sexy. Listen, I know how hot it can be to hear "You're so wet." But wetness doesn't always equate to being down to fuck, because of something called arousal nonconcordance. While those with penises have a 50 percent overlap between arousal and how genitals respond (meaning their erections indicate that they are aroused), in those with vulvas, this drops to 10 percent, meaning that someone with a vulva may get wet looking at something sexually relevant (like porn) even though they're not into it or aroused. Wetness or an erection are the body reacting to what may be seen as something that could be sexually relevant, basically. But arousal isn't just your body being aware of something sexual; it's also when you *expect and enjoy* the erotic simulation. Arousal nonconcordance tells you to *listen to your mind and to your partner's mind.* Just because someone is wet or erect doesn't mean they're turned on. If you've used this as a gauge of how hot and heavy things are getting, this can feel disappointing to find out. But what it means is that you have the chance to communicate to your partner and to listen in turn. This also means that *not* being wet doesn't mean you're not horny as fuck. It might just mean it's time for lube. Want to know if someone's turned on? Ask, and adjust accordingly.

MYTH 5: YOUR FANTASIES ARE UNHEALTHY

One of the tenets of sacred sexuality means liberating your erotic inspiration, your fantasies, and your imagination, and following these trails to evolution and sacred transgression. You may have been told that your fantasies are dirty, but actually they are healthy and normal! Far from being something to be ashamed of, they are reflections of your sexual health. In fact, sexual fantasies are so common, "it's actually considered pathological *not* to have sexual fantasies" (emphasis my own). Science has recently shown that those who have sexual fantasies "have more sex, engage in a wider variety of erotic activities, have more partners and masturbate more often."

Your fantasies also reflect your needs. In this way, they can act as a tool of inquiry, helping you explore what it is you can invite more of in your life, whether it's connection, sensuality, transgression, or love. Your fantasies can be road maps of your exploration, acting as a subconscious guide into your exploits. Or . . . they can totally not be. You may have fantasies that are so intense they scare you—like rape fantasies, for example, which 62 percent of women report having—that you may never wish to act out. Or you may want to examine them in a ritualized, consensual context, called a "scene" in BDSM. You may have fantasies you want to reenact and dive into (which I like to think of desires), and some you don't (which continue to be just fantasies). Fantasies can be used for inspiration for ritual; as a way to get closer to your partner by revealing, reveling in, and sharing your desires; and as a path to understanding your subconscious longings with more compassion and clarity.

MYTH 6: ORGASM IS THE END GOAL

Orgasms are amazing. In the moment of pure pleasure, your ego dissolves for just a second and you're able to connect with the totality of existence. Orgasms are powerful portals—to the beloved, to the Divine, to true consciousness—but focusing on them as the ultimate goal can deter the presence necessary for sacred sex to reach its fullest potential. You know the saying, "a watched pot never boils"? Thinking about and obsessing over orgasm is more likely to make you stressed out because you're so dependent on that "thing" to happen, and that stress stops you from getting aroused and being in the moment. Sacred sex is a journey, not a destination. Orgasms are wonderful, and they will more than likely happen a fair share of times during your exploration. But they are not the goal. Even when you're raising sexual energy to charge a working, you don't need one to be effective.

For survivors of sexual trauma especially, rushing for the big O may not be what's needed at all. Sacred sex is about so much more than penetration. It's about coming back to the body and the pleasures it brings—but there's no rush to get here. Certified sex therapist and award-winning author Stefani Goerlich encourages survivors to start slow. "Sexual trauma can often result in somatic (body-based) trauma responses that might not come up immediately after the assault; so it's important to give yourself time to gently explore the terrain of your body, and identify any new potential sensitivities," she shares. "Spending time touching your naked body, remembering that it is yours, and paying close attention to how it responds to various kinds of touch, is an important part of this healing process."

THE PATH OF PLEASURE AND ECSTASY

In the world of sacred sex, pleasure is a sacrament. One of the most important aspects of walking this path is knowing what you value, what brings you pleasure, and what the erotic means *to you*. Of course, this will be influenced by those in your life who help you open and evolve sexually, but ultimately it's you who's the judge of what the erotic, the sensual, and the pleasure-filled mean.

Pleasure happens in the brain and nervous system. When you feel something pleasurable, either through drugs or sex or the senses, neurotransmitters such as dopamine are released into different parts of the brain. The amount of dopamine released depends on context, culture, history, and biology, meaning that while you may get a huge hit from drinking red wine, someone else may get none. What this means is that once again, what feels good is personal. That said, all experiences of pleasure are related to the same brain system: fundamental pleasures such as food and touch, and higher-order pleasures such as money, music, and ecstasy all trigger the same parts of the brain. *Pleasure is literally wired in.*

Even thinking about a moment of pleasure can trigger this same system—a testament to the power of the brain. And while pleasure happens in the body, it's ecstasy that transports pleasure from something personal to something interpersonal, taking it out of the nervous system into the cosmic and something greater than yourself.

That's ecstasy. The path to ecstasy is paved with perverted intention, or good intentions, or sexy-as-fuck intentions. It can really be whatever you want because there are infinite paths to it.

REDEFINING THE EROTIC

One of the easiest ways to expand pleasure through self-knowledge is to create your own definitions for the words you'll be seeing and working with throughout this book. You already know how reductive and honestly *boooorrrrinnnggggg* it is to define sex as the penetration of a vagina with a penis. That leaves out about 95 percent of the body, and 75 percent of sexual acts that can bring just as much—or even more—pleasure than penetration alone. When you consciously redefine sex as something that serves your own relationship with it, such as "anything that has the potential to bring me full body pleasure" or "anything with the potential to bring me to orgasm," you expand into vast possibilities. In your grimoire, take some time to journal on the following. Feel free to turn this into ritual with some candles, mood lighting, tea, and the like. Invite in the possibilities of pleasure. Do an LBRP or a grounding and centering if it's in your practice. Invite in a God/dess of Love or Sex. Call upon your higher sexual self. Pull tarot cards, or conjure an erotic archetype for yourself and then begin.

Allow rewriting these definitions to be a starting point. You can write poetry, play or listen to music, read erotica or erotic poetry, dance and move your body, paint, pray, or do whatever else you need to do to channel pleasure into your words. Remember that these definitions aren't stagnant, and that as your journey with sacred sex transforms, so will your relationship to these words.

HOW DO YOU DEFINE . . .

Sex

E.g.: Anything with the potential to help me experience pleasure and/or to get me off.

Sensuality

E.g.: The way I embody a sense of pleasure and desire within myself. My relationship with pleasure and desire in relation to how I move through the world.

The erotic

E.g.: My personal relationship to that which invites in experiences of transcendent pleasure through a current of desire. The embodiment, experience, and interaction of that which stimulates, entices, and invites in sexual pleasure. My natural state of being.

Conscious sex

E.g.: A full-bodied approach to the sexual rooted in presence and connection with self/the beloved/the Divine. A way of showing up that honors my fullest erotic and spiritual expression, so I may be seen as a sacred vessel.

Sacred sexuality

E.g.: A framework for life that is based in the innate power of the erotic as fuel for magick, pleasure, evolution, ecstasy, and gnosis. A spiritual path that emphasizes immanence by accepting and reveling in the divinity of life, especially that of the body.

Pleasure

E.g.: That which enlivens me and takes me to the edges of self, where I can surrender to and be held by the Divine. That which brings me to a state of full-bodied bliss.

Ecstasy

E.g.: That which transcends pleasure as being solely of the body and elevates this to a full body and spirit experience. Pleasure that is rooted in something larger than myself, where I feel it fully and completely and am Divinely enveloped in it.

SACRED SEX AND MAGICKAL CHILDREN

Ascribing to the power of magick means anything that happens on the physical plane has an effect on the energetic planes, and vice versa. That's why when you cast a spell, the energies move from the energetic realms of existence down into the physical realms of existence. This same idea is why cleaning your home and cleansing your body have an effect on the spiritual plane. Everything is connected. In this way, when you are performing acts of sacred sex, especially with a partner, you are birthing something into the world through the release of energy and sexual fluids. This is often called a "magickal childe" and is part of the reason sex magick is so effective. An orgasm, or the release of an intense amount of sexual energy, moves into the world, and when it's impregnated with an intention, it can germinate and grow before becoming a reality.

I'm not talking about some demon spawn (although you can fuck demons; check out *Sex, Sorcery, and Spirit* by Jason Miller). A magickal childe isn't going to come and fuck up your life and ask you for all your money, unless you're not practicing safe sex and have a real child who grows up to ask you for things. A magickal childe is a way to perceive and think of the energies you're creating through sex as *creative and fertile energies with the potential to bring new things into this world*. While you can practice sacred sex with the intention of conceiving a human child who's also a magickal childe or moonchild, I'm referring to a seedling of something new that *will* manifest physically. This could be a house, a book deal, a magickal practice or path, or a shifted perspective. It could be a relationship, a lover, or an artistic muse. Your magickal childe will, if done right, be the manifestation of your intention. It's sex magick, baby!

SAFE SEX: IRL AND IN SPIRIT

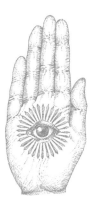

Being a devotee of the flesh means honoring the sexual with wisdom and integrity. This means practicing safe sex, both physically and spiritually. Since sacred sexuality requires honesty, communication, and trust, it's vital. To practice safe sacred sex means doing what you need to do in the physical realm to have all your bases covered so when it comes time to do the fun stuff, there's not a worry left in your mind to focus on. Condoms? Available, plentiful, and enchanted. STD/STI status? Known and agreed upon. Energetic and etheric body? Centered, protected, and grounded. Heart? Open and ready. Boundaries? Negotiated. Mind? At ease, and ready to be turned the fuck on.

Safe sex in the physical realm means getting tested regularly for sexually transmitted diseases and infections (STDs and STIs). It means being honest about having any viruses such as HIV, human papillomavirus (HPV), or herpes. It means using condoms and other forms of contraception and protection like birth control. It means keeping in mind that you can't use oil-based lubes with latex condoms or they could break.

Safe sex in the spiritual realm means coming to the temple centered. It means cleansing yourself of any negative or heavy energies. It means keeping an honest and open spirit, ready to show up fully in your power. Safe spiritual sex also can mean things like enchanting your condoms and birth control for extra protection or your lube with your intention. It means connecting with your Gods, your Holy Guardian Angel, your True Will.

The crossover of physical and spiritual safe sex is *communication*. If you can't communicate your STD/STI status, or even ask your partner about this, how do you expect to communicate your desires, much less about the sex you're having as you're having it? I know how scary it can be to ask about test status, or to share the fact that you live with something like herpes, HIV, or HPV. There's so much stigma around sexually transmitted anything, and the ingrained shame runs deep. But part of the work of the sacred sex Priest/ess or magician is unraveling this shame. Part of the spiritual work here is showing up without guilt around your past or around your health. You are doing your best, and having an STD or STI doesn't make you "dirty." Erasing the dichotomy of "clean" or "dirty" around STD/STI testing is part of the work. *Your test didn't come back clean or dirty; it came back positive or negative.*

A CONDOM BLESSING

You may use this simple charm to help enchant your condoms with extra protection. You can also do this over any form of birth control, changing *condom* to *birth control*.

Before you begin, have one partner place a hand under the condom and then place the other partner's hand on top of this. Then both hold one palm over the condom. Breathe, and feel yourself drawing Divine, healing, protective, white light from the cosmos above, through the crown of your head, through your spine and body, down your arms, and out your palms. Feel this white protective light infusing the condom. Stay in this visualization as long as you need, and when you're ready, repeat the following out loud:

> *I bless this condom with protection*
> *In the name of Divine indiscretion*
> *May it help us stay safe in all ways always*
> *From the physical to the highest spiritual plane*
> *And so it is.*

Once you're finished, you may use your condom. Repeat and enjoy.

SELF-LOVE AND SELF-LUST
AS SACRAMENTS

One of the most revolutionary moments in my relationship to my sexuality came when I was in a place of deep loneliness. I was longing for a partner to love and desire and lust over me in a way I had never been loved, desired, or lusted over. This came as I was discovering BDSM, when I was just opening up to the wide world of kink and fetish, and beginning to uncover my own desires and my sexuality. Because my introduction to this world was through a partner I was no longer seeing, I felt lost, like I had been exposed to a great secret, a new part of myself, but the door had been swung shut before I could even get my foot inside. I felt teased, alone, tormented, and insatiable.

This shifted one day when I realized that to have someone give me what I desired, I had to give it to myself first. To welcome the kinky magick I so desperately wanted, I had to find ways to *bring it into my life by myself.* This aha moment, when I realized to get the lover I so desired, *I had to become my own lover,* kick-started a yearlong journey of self-exploration.

What I didn't realize at the time was that years later, I would find the words to describe this ethos, and that I would continue to live it as a path of my exploration, even after I did begin to find partners who allowed me to adventure into the uncharted territories of my flesh. This ethos, as I have come to call it, is *self-lust.*

Many of you are probably familiar with—and practicing already— self-love, the sister of self-lust. Though self-love has become a commercialized cliché, it is still a powerful form of self-worship and self-care. Self-love is when you give yourself the adoration, support, compassion, and care you long for. Self-love means going to therapy as much as it does honoring your boundaries as much as it does relaxing in a bath with a joint after a long day. It's when you make your bed, brush your teeth, and shower. It's any form of self-care paired with an offering of wholeness from the heart. Sacred sex practiced solo is often a huge form of self-love, served with a heaping side of self-pleasure. It's the modern-day independent anthem that says "I can get myself off, and usually the results are much better than having mediocre casual sex with someone who doesn't bother to ask or care about my desires."

Self-lust is the kinkier, more provocative, and subversive older sister of self-love, and it is one of the pillars of this book. *Self-lust is finding sexual pleasure, excitement, desire, and longing within the self and for the self.* Unfortunately, organized religion has really tried to ruin a lot for those who walk any sort of path of sacred sexuality, and the idea of lust is no different. The Catholic Church defines lust as a "disordered desire for or inordinate enjoyment of sexual pleasure. Sexual pleasure is morally disordered when sought for itself, isolated from its procreative and unitive purposes." Fortunately, for those of you who are perverts like me, this definition against the sexual pleasure of the flesh probably only inspires you to enjoy it all the more. Because if the Catholic Church says it's bad, then it's sure to feel really, really good.

Self-lust means feeling hot and horny for your darkest truths, for your most intimate and vulnerable desires. It means accepting who you are as a way of personifying the Divine Erotic. On the next pages, find some ways to begin exploring self-lust. There will be many spells, rituals, practices, journal questions, and affirmations to follow, so use the following as a starting point. Then use the affirmations and prompts to supplement what you've read and worked with.

HOW TO BEGIN CULTIVATING SELF-LUST

- Figure out what styles, looks, and aesthetics make you feel sexy. Figure out what makes you feel turned on by your own damn self—and then find ways to wear it just for you. If you work from home, wear a sexy outfit during the day. Or if you usually just hang out in last night's pajamas and sweatshirt in the evening, try dressing up in something that makes you feel hot hot hot. Look in the mirror as often as you can, and enjoy whatever feelings come up. Creating desire for yourself is a part of this work.

- Once you figure out what you feel sexy in, take selfies and self-portraits in that. It may take a while to figure out what posing and angles work for you, but it's worth it. Capturing your glamour, power, and beauty, and saving the evidence for a low-self-esteem day is everything.

- Seduce yourself. When you pass a mirror, wink. When you go to brush your hair, do so in an enticing manner. As you put on perfume or cologne, imagine you're doing so for a lover—but the lover is *you*. Do a solo strip tease as you put on or take off your clothes. Put on your favorite lipstick or tie. Wear those jeans that make your ass look amazing. Say sexy things into the mirror. All of these concepts feel basic but aren't as easy. The more comfortable you get with your sexuality, the easier it will be to be fed by your own erotic essence.

- Spend time at your altar meditating on your sexuality. Write yourself a letter; pray about your own exploration of the transgressive; or simply decorate, clean, and cleanse your sacred space as an offering to your lust.

- See your body as an altar of lust, and treat it as such. When you masturbate or have sex, that's an offering to the lust you hold within yourself. Put your pleasure first. Allow yourself to get lost in self-seduction, honoring your body and whatever it is that it brings up for you.

- Weave your sexuality into your day-to-day life. This can mean talking to your friends about sex and the erotic, but it also means allowing yourself to be turned on by life. The more ways you're able to infuse your seductive creativity and awakening into your everyday life, the more you'll be able to feel the expansiveness of lust. Allow the wind on your cheek to feel like a touch from a lover, or the smell of the rain to tingle and resonate through you. Allow eye contact from a stranger to lead you into a land of awakening possibility, igniting a well of desire within you.

TRAUMA-INFORMED PRACTICES TO HELP YOU BEGIN REENGAGING WITH YOUR SEXUALITY

One of the things I want to remind you of is that there is no rush. Everyone's journey is unique. This is even more true if you're a survivor of sexual trauma of any kind. If your relationship with sexuality changed after your assault, you're not alone. Caring for yourself as you are right now is a deep act of kindness, self-compassion, and self-love. Find some simple rituals in the following pages to help you reengage with your sexuality as you see fit. Many of these were inspired by my dear friend Isabella Frappier, who is a sexual activist and trauma-informed pleasure mentor, focused on body literacy and sexual sovereignty.

- *Work with a Goddess of pleasure and love like Venus, Aphrodite, or Hedone.*

  Not everyone has access to a support system, like a therapist or friend who understands what you're going through. If you want cosmic assistance on your healing journey, you may wish to work with a face of the Divine Feminine like Venus, Aphrodite, or Hedone, who are Goddesses of sensual and sexual pleasure. These Goddesses can help you "reclaim pleasure as your birthright, and to really have the support of a Matron or an angel that you want to work with to hold you in that practice," Frappier shares with me. They invite you to see the Divine Erotic in everything, even that which is not sexual by nature: washing your hands, finding a new artist you love, or the smell of a blooming flower. Create an altar for a Goddess of your choice (adapting the instructions on pages 41–43), or spend a certain amount of time in a devotional to one of them (adapting the instructions on pages 218–24).

- *Give yourself permission to stop.*

  One of the things that sex therapist Stefani Goerlich emphasizes is how important it is to honor what you're feeling in the moment. "Give yourself permission to stop if necessary. Sometimes, simply knowing that you have the power to choose is enough to reduce our activation," Goerlich explains to me. However, if you find yourself engaging sexually and begin to feel overwhelmed but are called to continue, ground in your body without leaving the scene. "Pick a single sense to focus on: smell and touch are great to start with. Pay close attention to everything you can smell: your skin, your partner's sweat, the aroma of your bodies, the scent of the bedding. Try to identify each individual smell you can, then move on to another sense and repeat the exercise. This allows you to ground yourself within the scene, rather than stepping out of it," she says.

- *Work with the Moon.*

As a result of trauma, Frappier explains, menstruating humans can have their cycles turned all topsy-turvy. "That can make you feel really off-kilter and at least for me, uncertain of my place in the world spiritually. So it can really help to have some kind of structure that holds your practice," she suggests. One such structure is working with the lunar cycles. You can take note of what phase and sign the Moon is in every day and ask yourself how this feels in your body. Keeping a journal, alongside noting when the full and new Moons are, can benefit when it comes to tracking your healing. You may also check out the section on erotic lunar magick on page 201 for further guidance.

- *Work with the personification of time, like through Saturn or Binah.*

If working with the lunar cycles seems too etheric, try working with time as personified by Saturn, at the suggestion of Frappier, or through the Qabalistic energy of Binah. Personifying time can help you work through grief and trust in the healing process. It's not that it will go away, Frappier explains, but it will morph and become easier to deal with. Like working with a Goddess, working with the natural force of time as personified by a god or energy can help you talk to it, communicate with it, and understand it more fully.

• *Work with the ocean.*

The ocean's cyclical existence, its low and high tides, and its beauty make it a great muse for healing and releasing anything that's hindering it. One of my favorite rituals to practice in real life or meditation is one that Frappier also suggested to me. Bring flowers to the ocean, either solo or in community, and imbue them with everything you want to release and let go of through a moment of breath, meditation, or mindfulness. When you're ready, throw them into the ocean, trusting her to take what you're offering and release it. You can also perform this as a visualization in meditation if you don't have access to the ocean.

JOURNAL QUESTIONS

You've done plenty of unlearning and relearning when it comes to sex ed. Now it's time to put this in the context of conscious sexuality that works for you. Writing it all the hell down is a great way to start. As always, I invite you to turn your journaling session into as much of a ritual as you want, following the steps laid out in the first chapter. Remember, you don't have to answer every question. Pick the ones that resonate (or the ones that completely don't and inspire you to dig past your comfort zone), and see where they lead you. There are no right or wrong answers.

• What are the myths around sexuality you grew up with? Which do you still believe? How can you begin to release and let go of them?
• Using your own definition of sex, when was the first time you

experienced this? How does this new definition alter your experience, if at all?

- What are your favorite sexual fantasies? Which are the ones you hope to one day make a reality? Which are the ones you hope stay just as fantasies?
- How does taking the pressure off of orgasms help you be more present during sex? How does this bring an even greater sense of pleasure into your experience, if at all?
- What does pleasure mean to you? How does this differ from ecstasy?
- How can you invite more pleasure and ecstasy into your sex life and mundane life?
- How do you practice safe sex in the physical realm? In the spiritual realm?
- What makes you feel safe and cared for during sex?
- What does self-love mean to you? Self-lust?
- How can you cultivate more self-lust in your own life? How can you infuse this into your day-to-day life?

A TAROT SPREAD FOR AWAKENING SELF-LUST

As a complement to the journal questions, I invite you to pull tarot or oracle cards around self-lust. Allow these cards to speak to you symbolically, taking the time to write down what you see in your Sacred Sex Grimoire. You may not understand the answers you receive right away, but understanding will come with time. This three-card spread will help you gain perspective around the ways you can infuse the Divine Erotic into your own rituals of self-care. After setting up your space, ground and center, and begin to breathe. As you shuffle the cards, hold your intention in mind, whether that's something specific or as simple as, "How can I invite more self-lust into my life?" When you feel called, split the deck, pull your cards, and record the results alongside your interpretations.

Card 1: Where in my life can I invite in more self-lust?
Card 2: How can I embody and awaken this?
Card 3: How can this inspire my exploration of sacred sex?

AFFIRMATIONS

Work with these affirmations to remind yourself that you get to dictate what sexuality and Eros mean to you. Use them to remind yourself of your own erotic appetites, to affirm your new and supportive beliefs, and to release those that are keeping you from stepping into your power. These affirmations can support your journey to the sacred sex life of your most divinely perverted fantasies. Follow the guidance in Chapter 1 for creating a practice with affirmations that supports you.

- I expand all possibilities of pleasure.
- I redefine sex to serve my desires, myself, and my needs.
- I get to define what pleasure and sex mean to me.
- My body is divine, perfect, and erotic as fuck just as it is.
- I share my sexual boundaries clearly, with confidence and grace.

- I allow pleasure to course through me, and I experience this fully in my body.
- I am guided by magick and pleasure in all I do.
- I redefine the erotic on my own terms, to suit my own path.
- I bring forth the magick I desire into the world through love, sex, and Eros.
- I honor myself by practicing safe sex in all planes, in all ways, always.
- Sacred sex guides me toward creativity and a deeper sense of self.
- I am protected by my boundaries and grounded in my desires.
- I cultivate self-lust within myself with a sense of play, purpose, and self-seduction.
- Self-lust guides me deeper into my own erotic essence.
- I am my own favorite lover.

A SPELL TO ACTIVATE SELF-LOVE AND SELF-LUST

This spell is meant to be worked with solo because it's an activation spell of self-lust and self-love. These are foundational aspects of *your* relationship with sacred sexuality, even if you are already in sacred relationship or have a sacred sex/sex magick partner.

This ritual utilizes journaling, rose medicine, candle magick, and sexual energy to awaken your own powers of love, lust, and Eros. You will be left with a charged, consecrated, and anointed candle to light whenever you engage with sacred sex.

The rose is an emblem of magick and the mysteries of love and sex. Roses are sacred to Venus Aphrodite, Babalon, Mary Magdalen, Mother Mary, Oshun, and Isis, among other Goddesses. They are both beautiful and protective; their sweet scent and blooming petals are welcoming, while their thorns are an omen of strength, protection, and resilience. The rose displays both effervescent beauty and vulnerability and a powerful defense system. So, too, do self-love and self-lust require radical vulnerability and heart opening while also calling for strong boundaries.

In this ritual, you will be working with an adapted form of the Qabalistic Cross, which aligns your will with that of the Divine/cosmic/source.

What you need: A seven-day pull-out jar candle in red, orange, pink, or white (with its glass jar); oils like olive oil, la flamme oil, Venus oil, or honey; and herbs like cinnamon, dried rose petals and/or thorns, jasmine, passion flower, blue lotus, or glitter to dress the candle; tools, a pen, or a pencil to carve your candle; your Sacred Sex Grimoire and a pen or pencil; a red rose; any sex toys and lube you want to work with; and any crystals, tarot cards, or divination tools that can be placed on your altar near your candle or held as you practice sex magick.

This ritual is best done at the new, waxing, or full Moon.
It is especially potent on Friday, the day of Venus,
when all matters of love and lust are supported.

Before you begin, you may consecrate yourself and your space with sacred smoke. Also cleanse your candle, the jar it comes in, and whatever else you'll be using. You may use frankincense and myrrh (sacred to Goddesses of Love like Isis and Venus) or rose incense. If you're working with a resin like frankincense or myrrh, light a piece of activated charcoal, wait until it's all lit, and then place some resin on top, or just light the incense or dried rose petals, blowing out the flame so there's smoke. Then work with this smoke by fanning it around yourself, your space, and the objects you want to cleanse, visualizing any negative energy leaving. You can perform divination to gain clarity around the outcome of this ritual before you begin using tarot or oracle cards. If you have an erotic deck, this may be a great time to use it.

Step 1: Set up the space, ground, and shield

Set up your space, ground, and shield. If it's in your practice, you may perform the LBRP or the LBRH, or call in the elements and watch-towers. You may also cast your circle if you walk it.

Once you feel the Divine energy from heavens above you and the earth below you meeting and extending from your heart, you may call in your higher erotic self. This is the erotic archetypal power available to you at all times, guiding you and holding you in all you do. You may say something like the following, or write an invocation for yourself:

> *I call upon my higher sexual self, my most sensual self, my erotic truth, to guide me in this ritual of activating the powers of self-love and self-lust within me. May I be guided by forces and energies that work in my highest favor, in 100 percent light, so I may stand firmly in my sensual power, as I am meant to. And so it is.*

After you call upon this aspect of yourself, take a moment to breathe forth this energy from the highest realms of the cosmos into your body.

Step 2 (optional): Call in any deities or guides
Call in any deities or spirit guides you work with that can support this ritual. Let them know your intention—to activate the energies of self-love and self-lust as guides on the path of sacred sexuality—and ask for their support and blessings.

Step 3: Write a list of what you love and lust about yourself
Get out your Sacred Sex Grimoire, and write a list of what you love and lust about yourself. Write as many as you want in each category, aiming for at least ten in each, starting with *I love* _____ *about myself* and *I lust over my* _____, or whatever phrasing feels powerful as hell.

Remember that you are your harshest critic. Try to see yourself as a lover or friend would. Be compassionate. And remind yourself that self-love and self-lust don't have to be about physical traits. You can love your laugh and your sense of humor. You can lust over your desire to seek life to its fullest. You also can love the way your legs help you move and dance or lust after the shape of your breasts or penis. This is not the time to hold back and be humble, but to be proud and grateful.

Once you've written your list, take a moment to read it over and sit with it, making any adjustments you need.

Step 4: Read your list out loud, and charge and dress your candle
Hold your candle as you read your list of self-love and self-lust *out loud*, as this vibration will activate its energies into existence.

Dress your candle by carving and anointing it. You may pick a word that represents what you love about yourself and a word to represent what you lust about yourself. Use your tool, pen, or pencil to carve the words into the candle. You may also simply write "self-love" and "self-lust." Dress your candle with herbs and oils of your choice, rubbing from the ends into the middle of the candle or from the base up to the wick (both can draw something in), depending on what's in your practice. Then, sprinkle the herbs or glitter in this same way, or put some on a paper towel or plate and rub the candle in this.

Light the candle and say the following, rewriting or adapting as you see fit:

> On this day and at this hour, tapped into my fullest and most erotic
> power, I activate the energies of self-lust and self-love, brought
> forth from the highest and heavens above.
> May the Divine light descend to me and through me, to help me live
> and move forth in this energy,
> I align myself in will and heart, with the sacred powers of love and lust.
> This or something better for the highest good of all involved, and
> so it is.

Step 5: Call in self-love and self-lust, using the rose as a wand

Now you will tap into the powers and magick of the rose, using it as a wand to align yourself with the Divine and your fullest potential on the human plane, with a simplified version of the Qabalistic Cross. This ritual aligns your will, represented by a horizontal line drawn from shoulder to shoulder, with the Divine Will, represented by a line drawn from head to foot.

Hold your red rose in your right hand as you stand with your feet firmly planted, about hip width apart. Feel cosmic light from the heavens moving down to meet the crown of your head, and reach up with the rose as if you were drawing it down, touching the rose to the crown of your head. Then say the following:

From the highest heavens above

Trace a line down the front of your body with the rose, following your spine, and ending with the rose pointed at the ground next to your right hip, your arms straight down by your side. Then say the following:

To the deepest depths below

Hold the rose on your right shoulder. Then say the following:

On all planes

Now trace the rose across your heart and chest until it reaches your left shoulder, and say:

In all ways

Now hold your hands in prayer position at your heart with the red rose between them. Then say:

> *I align myself with the Divine Will and my own will to activate the energies of self-love and self-lust within me. May all past, present, and future versions of myself be steeped in this power fully. And so it is.*

Step 6: Sex magick
Grab any crystals that you wish to have around you. Caress yourself with your rose if you wish. As you inhale, feel your belly fill with air, and as you exhale, pull this energy up your spine, allowing it to rest

at the crown of your head and then repeat this. Once you've begun to circulate the sexual energy using the rose as inspiration and a guide, use sex magick to continue raising energy to charge your candle. Using whatever toys or instruments you'd like, begin to masturbate *while keeping the intention of cultivating self-love and self-lust in your mind*. You can even do this in front of a mirror. As you orgasm— or get as close as possible to orgasm—send this energy out through the crown of your head, into the cosmos, and into your intention, perhaps gazing at your candle as you do.

As you relax in the afterglow, tap into this energy of self-lust and self-love by visualizing yourself fully in its power. What would this *feel like*? How does it taste, smell, feel, and sound? What does it look like? Stay here, steeped in this visualization of your fullest sexual potential, for as long as you like.

Step 7: Close the ritual

When you're ready, find a comfortable position to close out the ritual, either sitting up or lying down. Notice how you feel and what the erotic energy in your body feels like. Take a moment to thank your higher sexual self, dismissing it and letting it know the ritual is finished, using the following or adapting or rewriting as you see fit:

> *I thank my higher sexual self, my most sensual self, my erotic truth, for guiding me in this ritual of activating the powers of self-love and self-lust within me. This working is done, and the activation is complete. I thank you for your guidance. You may leave with peace. So mote it be.*

If you invited in any deities or spirit guides, now is the time to dismiss them.

Perform the closing and grounding exercises.

If you invited in the elementals or watchtowers, now is the time to dismiss them. If you cast your circle by walking it, now is the time to close it. If you performed an LBRP or LBRH ritual at the beginning of the ceremony, now is the time to perform the Qabalistic Cross.

When you're done, you may press your forehead or the crown of your head into the ground, visualizing all excess energy making its way back into the crystal core of the earth.

*The candle you carved is one you will be lighting
again and again, any time you are exploring sacred sex,
or tapping into self-love and self-lust.
Snuff it out using a candle snuffer or fan, or by covering
the jar with thick fabric or the lid of a cauldron.
Relight it whenever you need, and when it's all finished,
you can dispose of it in a garbage can at a three-
or four-way intersection.*

CHAPTER 3

The Power of Sex Magick

You've officially entered the rodeo of the sex witch. Yee-haw, baby! You've jumped on the bull and begun to dissolve old beliefs around sex, and you've allowed yourself the power and pleasure of claiming your sexual energy as your own. Now you're going to learn how to further work with and manipulate this erotic power.

Sex magick is a way of changing the material world through the use of sexual energy, which is cultivated in the physical and etheric body and channeled for a desired purpose or intention. Sex magick = intention + sexual energy + action. It is a path of the erotic as a means of changing reality, and this can be done solo, with a partner, or with multiple partners. It is focused inward because the body becomes the wand, or the magickal instrument that directs the will of the individual into the cosmos for manifestation. It is only after your focus has gone inward—to circulating energy, to being present in pleasure and sensation, to connecting with the self or beloved—that you can turn your energy outward to cause real change. Sex magick may be practiced for the intention of knowing, cultivating, and expressing your sexuality in a more authentic way as well; it doesn't always have to be about manifesting.

In his book *Modern Sex Magick*, Donald Michael Kraig defines sex magick as "an ancient western system which sees the physical and non-physical as an interweaving continuum." I like this definition because of the way it explains the physical and nonphysical, which are both key components to sex magick as well as sacred sexuality. The physical (the flesh and genitals) acts as a portal to the nonphysical (the etheric body and energy, the heart, the soul). When these two aspects of self are worked with in union: magick.

One of the reasons sex magick is so powerful is because of the potency of the orgasm. (I want to note that those who live with anorgasmia can still practice sex magick even if orgasm isn't possible.) Orgasms open the gateway to the numinous. There's a reason the French call them *la petite mort* or "the little death." The mysteries of sex and death are one and the same. At the moment of climax, the rational mind becomes nonexistent, as if the gateway has opened to pure consciousness. It is this moment, when paired with an intention or desire, that makes sex magick so powerful.

Sex magick isn't just one practice or method, but a range of techniques that utilize sexual energy as a means of transformation. And while sex magick is a part of sacred sexuality, it's only one path. Sex magicians and sex witches may have a sacred view of sex, or they may not. They may see it as deserving of reverence, or just see it as another tool in their practice. You don't have to practice sex magick to live a life devoted to sacred sexuality, but if you're anything like me, these two aspects of the self are intertwined.

You can practice sex magick for an infinite number of reasons, just as you can practice magick for an infinite number of reasons. Here are just a few.

PEOPLE PRACTICE SEX MAGICK TO . . .

- Manifest a desired intention (money, a new job, more sex, more partners, a new home).
- Banish something (shame, external influences, bad habits or patterns).
- Connect with the Divine.
- Better know and engage with their etheric or subtle body.
- Better know and engage with their sexual energy and self.
- Find more confidence and comfort in their erotic selves.
- Raise sexual energy as a form of ritual, prayer, or offering.
- Charge or consecrate a talisman or amulet.
- Connect with energetic beings such as Goddesses or Gods, animal spirits, demons, or angels.
- Initiate themselves in a specific path or mysteries.
- Call forth something (creativity, inspiration, pleasure, or ecstasy).
- Send up a devotion to themselves, a deity, a path, or practice.

SEX MAGICK
AS WALKING THE LEFT HAND PATH

To walk the path of the sacred sex witch or erotic mystic is to embrace the Left Hand Path. The Left Hand Path (LHP) is an umbrella term for occult schools and philosophies that see the taboo, transgressive, and subversive as sacred. This means turning toward that which is rejected by mainstream society as a way of reclaiming the self. While sex isn't exactly rejected by Western society, those who use sex to gain power, or to claim their own, still are. This can be especially seen in the way sex workers are stigmatized, brutalized, and murdered at disproportionate rates. The LHP puts individual freedom and liberty above all else. This is a path of actualization through the self, not through the other.

The LHP can include working with sex, alcohol, drugs, and other substances as a means of invoking power and getting to know yourself, as in LHP tantra. The biggest difference between the LHP and Right Hand Path (RHP) is that the latter strives to *(re)unite* with the Divine, and to know the Divine, while those who follow the LHP strive to *become* the Divine through accepting and honoring pleasure and the senses, instead of rejecting them. Like everything else, the distinction between these two modalities isn't black and white (and the LHP isn't "black magick" or "evil," just as the RHP isn't "white magick" or "good"), and there are more subdivisions the further you go into any sect of magick or tradition. The good news is that you can work with both hands, and follow both paths, often called the Middle Way.

A BRIEF HISTORY OF SEX MAGICK

The practice of sex magick as we know it in the West didn't just appear out nowhere; it came about through the merging of philosophies and mystic traditions. The history of sex magick takes up volumes in its own right, but I wanted to highlight some of the most influential sex magicians for inspiration.

PASCHAL BEVERLY RANDOLPH

If you're familiar with sex magick, then you have Mr. P. B. Randolph to thank. The man, the myth, the legend introduced the very concept to the West. Born in 1825, Randolph was a free Black man raised in New York. A spiritualist, doctor, writer, and activist, he advocated for the rights of People of Color and women. Randolph authored the book *Magia Sexualis*, which was published fifty years after his death (and translated and amended by in/famous occultist Maria de Naglowska), and founded the Brotherhood of Eulis.

While erotic spirituality has been around for thousands and thousands of years—more than likely for as long as people have been fucking—Randolph created an organized system of spiritual sexuality that he called "Affectional Alchemy," and it is with him that we see a "detailed, sophisticated, and well documented" *system*. Randolph believed that sacralized sex was the key to true transformation, both on a worldwide scale and on a personal scale, and that his system of working with orgasms could open the door to magical powers and new spiritual realms—as if the orgasm was a portal to any wish, desire, or intention. To Randolph, sex magick was *the* life hack.

ALEISTER CROWLEY, THE MASTER THERION, THE GREAT BEAST 666

Paschal Beverly Randolph remains largely out of the erotic occult milieu, but the same cannot be said about the most infamous bad boy of the esoteric, Aleister Crowley. Known also as the Master Therion, the Great Beast 666, and "the most wicked man in the world," among other epithets, Crowley is probably the most influential occultist of the past three hundred years. When he was born in 1875, his mother gave him the nickname of the "Great Beast," inspired by the Book of Revelations, which later would influence his concept of the occult as well as his philosophical and magickal movement and religion known as Thelema. Crowley was introduced to the occult group the Hermetic Order of the Golden Dawn in 1898, and in 1899, he began to study Eastern traditions such as yoga and tantra.

It was in 1904 that Crowley received his greatest teaching, *The Book of the Law*, through a series of channeled messages using his wife, Rose Kelly, as a medium. This book is the holy book of Thelema, which is based on sexuality and erotic expression and the coming forth of a new spiritual aeon. Thelema posits the ritualistic breaking of societal taboos, including consuming sexual fluids, having sex with same-sex partners, and masturbation. Like the tantrikas, Crowley saw violating these taboos as a path to spiritual power.

Like Randolph, Crowley believed that sexuality was at the core of existence and had the power to change the world. Not only could it fuel magick, it also could destroy the ego, and *this* is the crux of Crowley's beliefs. The "ultimate transgression" for Crowley was using erotic energy and sex to shatter all preconceived ideas of the self, past a point of no return, which he calls "crossing the abyss." His vision of sex magick is carried forth through occult orders like the Ordo Templi Orientis, the A∴A∴ (which he founded), and Thelema, which states that "love is the law" and that "there is no law beyond do what thou wilt."

AUSTIN OSMAN SPARE

Austin Osman Spare (AOS) is the granddaddy of chaos magick—and an incredible and inspiring artist to boot. Born in London in

1886, Spare was involved with Crowley's A∴A∴ system of magick, but felt it was too constricting and tedious. Instead, he developed his own method of magick, and his own belief system, most notably his form of sigillary, the death posture, and the concept of Zos (the human mind) and Kia (the universal mind). At the core of Spare's belief and work was the idea that the subconscious mind is the truth, that it holds all the power to create and destroy—and that sexual energy is the way to crack this wide open. Labeled an "erotic magical diabolist" and a "satanic occultist," Spare was a boundary-breaking magician whose legacy is still felt today.

Spare, above all, was an artist who used drawing as his magickal medium, breaking out of any preconceived notions about what magick is meant to look like. He popularized a form of sigil-making that takes the letters from a statement of intention and uses them to create a symbol that is charged through masturbation. The basis of his philosophy, which can be found in his *Book of Pleasure*, is the idea of self-love and "sexual pleasure as the innermost nature of the self." Like Crowley, Spare believed sexuality shouldn't be denied but instead spread through pleasure. Spare used his art, magick, and the personal universe he created to express this, and his work was hugely influential to chaos magick that came after his time.

DION FORTUNE

Dion Fortune's impact on Western Esotericism is more profound in her work with the Qabalah than sex magick, but it still feels important to include her on this list. Fortune was born in England in 1890 and connected the concept of Divine light, or pure consciousness of the Godhead, with that of the libido. Like the concept of Kundalini in yoga, she saw sexual energy as life force energy, and its most powerful expression. Fortune's beliefs about sexuality changed as she went further on her path, and although she never was explicit about sexual magick, in her book *The Esoteric Philosophy of Love and Marriage*, she does talk about how energy raised during sexual intercourse can be collected or compressed and used or exerted, as energy raised during sex creates a vortex of power that extends up the planes, or energetic levels of reality. Fortune acted as a link between groups like the Ordo Templi Orientis (OTO) and the later pagan revival started in part by Gerald Gardner, and her work, nonfiction books, and novels continue to influence occultists today.

MARIA DE NAGLOWSKA

Satanic woman and esotericist Maria de Naglowska is another infamous figure in the history of sex magick. Born in 1883, Naglowska's psychic gifts were noted early, and she developed an interest in the esoteric while finding refuge in Rome after being imprisoned for her radical ideas. Over the years, Naglowska led salons and occult circles and gained a reputation for discussing Satanism and sex magick. Eventually, she founded *de la Confrérie de la flèche d'or*, or the Brotherhood of the Golden Arrow, in 1932, which shaped her beliefs about sex magick in relation to femininity. Naglowska envisioned a third aeon rising: the first was Judaism, or the age of the father; the second term was Christianity, or the age of the son; and the third would be of the holy spirit, or the mother, which was to be a sex magick and feminist utopia. Her most infamous ritual involved hanging and penetration while unconscious from this act.

GERALD GARDNER

Gerald Gardner was born in 1884 and is the creator of the modern neo-pagan religion Wicca. A nudist who developed the idea of performing ritual "skyclad" (or naked), Gardner said he was initiated into a New Forest, England, coven of witches whose beliefs and practices had been passed down for thousands of years. While this is apocryphal, Gardner is one of—if not *the*—fathers of the pagan revival movement in the 1960s, thanks in large part to the publication of his book *Witchcraft Today* in 1954, only four years after Britain repealed its witchcraft laws.

A large part of Wicca is based on the Goddess, the female body, and the Priestess. Like occultists before him, Gardner believed in the power of sexual energy, which could be raised, contorted, and worked with through ritual, including that of sex and flagellation. To represent the sacred union of sexuality through the masculine and feminine, Gardner created—or ripped off from Crowley—the "Great Rite." The Great Rite is the sexual union (which can be literal or represented by a sword piercing a chalice) of the High Priestess and High Priest of the coven who epitomize and represent the joint ecstasy of the Goddess and the God. There are many similarities between Wicca and Thelema, one of them being that sex is the strongest and most immense magickal force there is.

COURTESANS

Now we turn to some of the icons who have defined the way society views the erotic: the courtesans. Courtesans reached the peak of their power in the Belle Époque in Europe, specifically Paris. They were often mistresses who were treated lavishly by nobility and royalty and were knowledgeable in art, fashion, food, and culture. I am including them in this list because they express a way of working with sexuality and enchantment through glamour and charm as a means to an end: riches.

They emulated Venus, the Goddess of Love, by taking the desires of their beloved and reflecting them as a sacred mirror. In fact, many of the nude or revealing paintings of Goddesses—including Venus— from the Renaissance are fashioned after courtesans, who had the liberty to show skin in a way other women didn't. Courtesans carried the current of the Goddess by holding a space of beauty, majesty, and

Sex Witches Support Decriminalizing Sex Work

Just a reminder! If you call yourself a sex witch, a sex mystic, or a practitioner of sacred sex in any shape or form, it's imperative that you also take the time to support the decriminalization of sex work. Legalization would put laws in place to make sex work and the act of selling sex something that is regulated and legal, but legalization leaves out the voices of sex workers themselves and their needs, instead reverting to what the state or country *thinks* is best, which is often whorephobia (or the fear and discrimination of anyone who profits off their sexuality) disguised under layers of law. The model that should be supported is decriminalization, which centers workers' rights, putting sex workers on the front lines in building legislation that the community wants and needs. With commercialized sex decriminalized, those in the industry can access labor laws—ones that actual sex workers, not civilians, helped put in place. Check out the "Resources" section at the back of this book for organizations and resources to help support decriminalization and the protection of sex workers.

grace for their lovers and the world who admired them. In short, courtesans turned themselves from object to subject, and in this way reclaimed their sexuality as a source of power. This is why they are part of the legacy of sex witches and sex magicians that you can tap into when you're summoning your own erotic essence.

EROTIC VOTARIES

Known more commonly as the sacred prostitutes of antiquity, erotic votaries were the priestesses who embodied the Goddess of Love at Her temple and served Her by engaging in ritual sex with those who came to worship. Priests also served the same function, exemplifying the role of God for those who wanted to worship. It is said that there were erotic votaries at the temples of Inanna and Ishtar in Mesopotamia and Babylon, for Venus and Aphrodite in Rome and Greece, and possibly even for Isis (or Auset) in Egypt, although the exact history is disputed. By seeing their partner as God, and by incarnating as the Divine Feminine, they created a shift in consciousness, exalting the sex act to a sacred one. When you engage with ritual sex or sex work, you're carrying forth the legacy of the erotic votaries.

A note: I use the term *erotic votaries* here and through this book to refer to sacred prostitutes because of the distinction that so many academic, texts, and historians create between "sacred prostitution" and "profane prostitution," or selling sex outside of the temple or ritual environment. I feel that "erotic votary" is a better choice to describe those who work with sex as a sacrament to the Goddess.

SEX MAGICK 101: THE BASICS

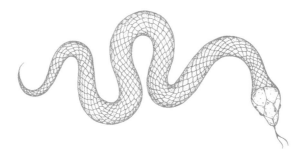

Sex magick doesn't have to be a part of sacred sex. You can bring cosmic and mystical consciousness to your sex life and never practice a spell or ritual. But my opinion is that you would be missing out. Remember: magick = action + energy + intention. A simple example is singing someone "Happy Birthday" as they blow out the candles on their birthday cake. The intention is simple—to wish them a joyous birthday and to invite blessings into this new year. The energy is raised through singing and holding space for this person, and the action is both the singing and the blowing out of the candles. That's a spell, baby! In this case, sex magick = action + intention + *erotic energy*.

If you are just beginning your sex magick practice, my suggestion is to work with the meditation on page 116 to begin feeling and moving sexual energy through your body. Then you can begin exploring sex magick when you masturbate. Sex magick can be performed solo or partnered, but my suggestion is to practice it alone if you're just dipping your toe into the smutty waters. This is because (1) knowing how sexual energy moves in your own body will help you understand what it feels like alongside someone else's sexual energy, and (2) having a solo relationship to sex magick will help you have a foundational understanding of what sacred sex means *to you*. Like any kind of sex, sex magick includes risk, both physical and energetic. Trust is the key that allows you to surrender to the ecstatic flow. It's much better to just DYY (do you yourself) in this case than it is to search Tinder for a partner because you think you need to.

Step 1: Set your intention

The first step in sex magick is knowing your why. Sexual energy is the energy of creation, and using it to manifest or bring something to you is a powerful choice. However, you also can use sex magick to banish something, as a way of transforming or purifying a situation, to connect to your sexual essence, as a form of devotion or offering to a deity or guide, or as a way to clear and cleanse your etheric body. Whether you're looking to find a new apartment, heal your body, offer energy to a Goddess of Love, banish negative self-talk and shame, or cleanse your body with the fire power of Eros, sex magick can be a potent tool.

Alongside setting the intention, you'll also want to decide if this is a solo or partnered practice.

Step 2: Set up the space, and make yourself feel hot AF

Now that you've decided on your intention, it's time to set up your space. But for sex magick, it also includes making sure you have the right toys, condoms, lube, and whatever else you need. This also means that you are creating an environment you *want* to fuck in. Be sure any dirty laundry is removed and that no pets or stuffed animals are staring at you—unless that's your thing. You can also use this time to work with correspondences. If you're channeling the fiery energy of Mars to banish negative self-talk around sex and love, you may want to decorate with the color red or burn five red candles or cinnamon or tobacco incense. If you're calling in self-lust and self-love, you may want to work with Venus and have fresh roses on your altar, seven green candles in the space, or rose quartz near the bed. Let your practice and path guide you.

Now you'll want to be sure that you feel hot as fuck. Use the process of adorning yourself as energetic foreplay. As you dress yourself, think of your intention and how incredible it's going to be as it manifests. Allow yourself to be seduced. If you're practicing sex magick with a partner or lover, connect with and crave each other. Wear something that makes you feel like a sex witch, or that you know your partner will want to tear off your body. You can wear perfume, cologne, and oil, but be sure it's not overwhelming—a couple sprays or dabs behind the ears and on the collarbone will suffice. If you're not afraid to get messy, red lipstick is always a sexy choice, but just beware: it will get absolutely everywhere.

You will be grounding and entering the temple, and you may wish to perform any preliminary rituals such as breath work now. If you're with a partner or partners, attuning your breath is a quick way to initiate intimacy. You may practice meditation, a banishing ritual, or invocation if you and/or your partners will be taking on the form of Godheads during your ritual. You may work with the Qabalistic Cross, or LBRP, or cast a circle and invite in the elements.

Step 3: Raise the erotic energy

Now comes the fun! Begin to masturbate or have sex and then choose your own adventure: (1) focus on your intention the entire time you are fucking and after, or (2) focus on your intention only at the moment before climax, during, and in the afterglow.

Enjoy the process. Next time, change it up from how you normally masturbate or have sex. Go slow, or go fast. Allow it to be sacred. Connect to your heart and your partner, *and don't forget to breathe*. Use your breath to move the sexual energy through your body, or to create a circuit of energy with your lover or lovers, sending the energy through your body and into theirs and having them do the same. You may wish to practice edging, pulling back as you feel yourself approaching orgasm, to continue raising energy.

Step 4: Focus on your intention as you get off, and send it to the cosmos
Once you feel yourself about to orgasm or as close as you can get, again focus on your intention if you haven't been the whole time. As you orgasm or feel the energy peak, feel it moving from your genitals, up your spine, through the crown of your head, and out to the cosmos. If you're working with a sigil, now is the time to focus on it and send it your energy. If you're having sex with a partner or partners and you don't orgasm simultaneously, allow whoever is orgasming to send out the energy and then turn their focus to their partner's orgasm, repeating the process of using breath, visualization, and focus to send out the energy through the body and into the universe.

Step 5: Visualize your desire in the afterglow
Enjoy the buzz coursing through your body as you visualize your desired outcome. Stay in the pleasure and what it would feel like for this intention or desire to be true, taking as much time as you need to do so.

Step 6: Close the ritual
Perform the grounding and closing exercises. Spend time now in aftercare—or prenegotiated postsex support—which can mean eating

chocolate, taking a bath, reading a book, or decompressing in any way you wish. If you did the LBRP or Qabalistic Cross before the ritual, now is the time to do another one to close it out. If you invoked a deity, now is the time to dismiss them. If you cast a circle and invited in the elements, close the circle and dismiss the elements. Now, forget all about your ritual and enjoy your newfound power as a sex witch.

The Ethics of the Sex Witch

One of the tenets of sex magick is knowing thyself. This means knowing your desires, knowing your limits, knowing your body, and knowing what your ethics are when it comes to sex magick. If you practice, or plan on practicing, sex magick with other people, then it's imperative that you start to figure out what you feel comfortable with. This means deciding if you need your partner(s) to know you're practicing sex magick with them (and receiving enthusiastic consent for this), or if you don't feel like you need to tell them what you're doing.

On one hand, consent is hot, and if you're raising energy during sex, the other person should probably know. On the other hand, if someone is already fucking you and consenting to that, how can they say no to whatever it is you're doing in your own inner world? This isn't black or white, and your beliefs around what feels right and doesn't will more than likely change depending on context and your practice. But taking the time to journal, explore, and excavate what you believe and feel comfortable with before you hit the sack will make it easier for you to honor your inner compass when it comes time for the sex magick itself. Use the following journal prompts to help guide you in this unraveling.

- Do I think it's necessary to tell my partner(s) I'm practicing sex magick? Do I think it's the right thing to do?

- If not, is it because I really don't see it as an issue, or because I'm scared they will say no and we won't be able to fuck?

- Would I want my partners to disclose this if they were doing it?

- What do my gut and my heart want me to know about this situation?

SIGILS AND SEX MAGICK

Sex happens in the body, but it also has roots in the unconscious and subconscious, which is one of the reasons that sex magick and sigils are such a powerful pairing. Sigils, popularized by the great magician Austin Osman Spare, are deconstructed intentions that are turned into symbols and then charged. The idea is that a sigil works as a container for a desire to unfold but through the subconscious. The conscious mind forgets what the sigil means and represents, allowing it to do its thing. *This is an integral part of the work.* For a sigil to be effective, its purpose and all details need to be forgotten as soon as the ritual is finished.

There are a couple of methods of working with sigils, but the premise is the same. You create your statement of intention and turn this into a symbol. The only difference is the way in which you engage with the sigil itself, either by making many and forgetting what it means before charging it, or by charging it immediately.

But first, why would you want to create a sigil? Well, sigils are easy, potent, and powerful magick. To be imprinted in the subconscious, they require you to be in an altered state of consciousness, one that includes a climax of energy, a crescendo. Because sexual energy naturally peaks, because sex naturally brings one to an altered state of mind, because sex is fun and easy, sigils and sex magick just work. Plus, you can charge a sigil *for any purpose* with sex magick—even for something as mundane as earning enough money to get your car fixed or finding the right doctor. So just know that these methods can be adapted for life outside your sacred sex practice as well.

REASONS FOR USING SIGIL MAGICK

- Protection of your sexual energy, of your space, or from those who have harmed you
- Banishing negative patterns around sex and the erotic, negative energy, old beliefs around sex, or guilt and shame
- Manifesting a new partner; a new relationship to your sexuality; a conscious relationship; kinky or sacred sex; or anything like money, a new apartment, or a job
- Deepening an existing relationship with sacred sex or turning a relationship into a conscious one
- Connecting to your sexual power and energy, dedicating your sexual energy to a deity, or consecrating a power dynamic or new relationship

METHODS OF SIGIL MAGICK

There are two main methods you can take when working with sigils. One is being aware of the sigil you're charging and using intention and visualization to empower your sigil before destroying it. The other is to make many sigils at once, leave them alone for a week so you forget what each means, and then charge them with sex magick one at a time over a specific time period. There are pros and cons to both methods.

On one hand, if you're aware of the sigil's intention, you can hold this in your mind as you perform the working and allow yourself to feel the desire. This can work wonders for something you feel intensely about. It is also a good choice if you need results ASAP. The downside is that this attachment and visualization can make it difficult to forget about the working and what the sigil represents. Thinking about the sigil after the fact, wondering if it's working, and sending it energy when the ritual is finished can undo all your work. You want to move on with your life to let the magick manifest as it should.

Instead, you can make a bunch of sigils at once, leave them in a bag or box, and come back to them days or weeks later. Pick a sigil to charge through sex magick, except instead of visualizing and feeling the outcome, just raise and direct energy to send to the sigil. You don't know what the sigil or ritual is for, and it's easier for your subconscious mind to do its thing without interference from your waking consciousness. If you don't have multiple goals you need a sigil for, or if you get easily distracted without something specific to focus on, multiple sigils might not be the best choice.

Try both methods and see what works for you. Your own preferences will guide you in what makes sense for your practice. Be flexible, take an approach that suits your vibe and energy, and trust the sigils will do the work.

CONSTRUCTING A SIGIL

Almost any ritual in this book can become more powerful with a sigil. Play around, see what feels right, and then record the results in your Sacred Sex Grimoire alongside any outcomes.

Here's how to construct a sigil:

* Set up your ritual space, ground, and shield.

* Use one of the aforementioned methods to create a statement of intention.

* Write this out and then cross out any repeating letters. You also have the option of crossing out vowels so you're left with only consonants. Try both and see which you like better. There's no "right" or "better" way.

* Take these letters and arrange them to form a symbol. The less the symbol looks like letters, the better. Try layering the letters, and let your imagination and the energy present dictate what comes next. You'll want to have a few pieces of paper to play around with different designs. Once you have a symbol you like, you can add flair like little lines at the ends (like a serif font).

* Draw a circle around the sigil so it becomes a container for your intention or desire.

* Depending on your method, make multiple sigils at once for different desires or intentions. Put them in a box or a bag, leave them somewhere where you won't see them for a few days or a week, and then pick one at random to charge.

- Charge the sigil through sex magick. As you masturbate or have sex, raise the energy to its peak, look at your sigil, and send it the energy as you feel yourself attaining your desire (if you know what your sigil is). When you're done (again, if you know the intention of your sigil), stay in the afterglow, feeling what it's like to have this as reality, noticing what it feels like to hold this within you.

- No matter if you know the intention of your sigil or not, destroy the sigil. You can burn it, rip it up and throw it out, bury it, or flush it down the toilet.

- Banish, laugh, clap, or stomp your feet as a way to close the ritual.

- Forget the working and why you made the sigil, and go about your day-to-day life. Let the magick do its thing, and you will be surprised at how intensely effective it is.

JOURNAL QUESTIONS

How does it feel to be a sex witch? Hopefully, you're feeling powerful as fuck and discovering new parts of yourself with each ritual or self-love session. This means it's the perfect time to unveil even more of your erotic power. Use these prompts as a guide, picking whichever ones resonate or trigger something, and allow them to guide you in your self-discovery, free writing, doodling, mind mapping, or poetry or prose writing. You can also use the accompanying tarot spread to go further. Turn it into as much of a ritual as you wish.

- What does sex magick mean to me?
- How does this inspire my relationship with the Divine Erotic?
- How do I define sex magick to resonate with my beliefs and spiritual practice?
- What erotic archetypes can I conjure to be grounded in my sexual power?
- What sex magicians of past or present inspire me? What sex icons, celebrities, or artists who I admire also carry this current?
- What is the creative expression I hope to carry with me?
- Do I plan on exploring sex magick solo or partnered? Both?
- How can I continue to support the fight for sex workers' rights and decriminalization?
- What does erotic and sexual energy feel like in my body? How do I recognize its presence? What awakens, activates, and triggers it?
- How does sex magick fit into my work with sacred sex?

A TAROT SPREAD FOR DIVING INTO THE DIVINE EROTIC

This spread will guide you further into your sex magick practice, with archetypal inspiration and knowledge about your practice. Use this to help find your inner compass, remembering the tarot reads where you are in the present moment and that it doesn't predict an unchanging future. Set up your space, your cards, and yourself. As you're ready, ask your question (which can simply be "How can I dive deeper into my sex magick practice?"), shuffle the cards, cut the cards if it's in your practice, and then pull your cards. When you're done, record your interpretations and any insight in your grimoire.

Card 1: What is my relationship to sex magick?
Card 2: How can I deepen it intentionally?
Card 3: Where can I look for inspiration?
Card 4: How can I bring this into my practice?
Card 5: How can I activate my sexual power?
Card 6: How can I carry this with me in all I do?

AFFIRMATIONS

These affirmations are here to hold you in your power. They are here to remind you of your strength. They are here to guide your practice and reflect to you your truth when you find it hard to remember. Use these as anchors during sex magick or to continue cultivating your sexual power. These will supplement the themes and explorations in this chapter, so take what resonates and leave the rest.

- I am divinely held and guided by my sacred erotic essence.
- I surrender to the current of sex magick within me.
- I connect to the lineage of sex magick on all planes, in all ways, always.
- I honor the magick of the Divine Erotic within me.
- I activate the magick of the Divine Erotic within me.
- I surrender to the power of my sexual magick.
- As I honor my magick, I move more deeply into my truth.

- I find power and magick in my erotic essence.
- I am a sex God/dess, and I embody my power through sex magick.
- I honor sacred sex as a path back to the Divine.
- I am an unstoppable sex witch.
- My magick and sexuality guide me into a life filled with pleasure and wonder.
- I'm a motherfuckin' sex God/dess.

A MEDITATION TO BEGIN FEELING SEXUAL ENERGY IN YOUR BODY

Energy is at the basis of magick of all kinds, and being able to recognize and feel it within your body is vital. Sexual energy is subtle, and it takes time and attention to begin to nurture, feel, and direct it. Meditation is one way to cultivate this awareness and will improve your ability to direct your sexual energy in spells and rituals.

Set up your space following instructions in Chapter 1. To begin, find a comfortable sitting position—in a chair with your feet against the earth, or on the ground with your legs folded. Take a moment to come back to your breath, moving more deeply into yourself with each inhale, and allowing all worries, anxieties, and tensions from the day to melt away with each exhale. As you feel a sense of inner stillness, breathe into and focus on your genitals or your sexual center, visualizing a fire here, and feeling as if each breath intensifies the flames. Stay here for at least five breaths, or as long as you can until the inner heat gets too intense. Then visualize this flame rising toward your heart center, where you see a chalice full of water. The fire begins to heat it, and with each breath, you feel this chalice get hotter and hotter, causing the water inside to boil and turn to steam. This feels erotic and expansive, and you stay here for at least five breaths or until you can't take the heat. Then, feel this steam rise until it reaches the crown of your head, where it turns into golden light and pure energy. With each breath, feel this energy strengthening and intensifying. Stay here for at least five breaths or until you feel like this energy is going to explode. Feel this light pouring forth from the crown of your head, flowing over your body, and pooling at the sexual center of your genitals, where it's absorbed into the fire and the process starts again. Feel this flow of energy move up and through you for as many cycles as you wish.

Once you recognize this energy, you can simply move it through your sexual center, your heart, and the crown of your head without visualizing the flames or chalice. Practice it in seated meditation and again when you're masturbating. Notice how it feels different when you work with sexual stimulation, and record in your grimoire what comes up.

Customizing Your Sex Magick Rituals

Throughout this book, you will have the option of working rituals solo, with a partner, or with partners. Please keep in mind that customizing your practice is always available to you even if, for the sake of avoiding repetition, I don't say so every time.

A SEX MAGICK RITUAL
TO CALL FORTH YOUR FULLEST
SEXUAL POTENTIAL AND POWER

Self-lust and self-love laid the foundation, and now you are committing to the path by living what it means to be a (sacred) sex witch. This means grounding into your erotic potential, actively choosing to see the ways in which the current of sexual energy can find its way into your mundane and magickal life. To live this path, and not just walk it occasionally, means finding the erotic within everything. This spell will mark this transition and rite of passage in a supportive and sensual way.

What you need: Any sex toys and lube you want, your grimoire and a pen or pencil, a tarot deck or card to represent the sexual power you wish to call forth, and your sacred sex candle.

This ritual is best worked during a new, waxing,
or full Moon because it's activating and draws in energy.

Step 1: Set up the space
Before you begin, per usual, you'll want to have your space set and your supplies gathered. This is a good time to set up your altar with anything you feel represents your intention for this ritual. You may also clean and cleanse your space and supplies, using sacred smoke or holy water or rose water.

Step 2: Set your intention

Take the time to set an intention in your grimoire. It may be to unleash your erotic potential, or you may have something unique or personal that you want to commit to. Now is the time to write it down clearly so you know what you're focusing on. Once that's done, pick an affirmation or word to work with that represents your intention. It can be something like, "I am ready to awaken the Divine Erotic within me" or a word like *awaken*. You will be anchoring your intention with this word or phrase as you work with glamour and adornment in the next step and during the sex magick portion of this ritual. If you are doing this ritual with a partner or partners, you can each have your own affirmation and intention to work with, or you may pick one as a couple.

Step 3: Get yourself ready through glamour and affirmations

As you slip into (or out of) something that embodies your erotic essence, notice the sensations, scents, and feelings that resonate with the energy of the ritual. *As you feel the energy shifting, come back to your affirmation or word of power.* Repeat it to yourself out loud. Allow it to guide you.

Wear something that makes you feel grounded in your sexual power and erotically unstoppable. If you're getting ready alongside a partner or partners, allow it to be a dance of seduction as well.

Step 4: Ground and call in

Now is the time to set up the space energetically and light your charged sacred sex candle. You may wish to perform the LBRP, practice chanting or drumming, cast a circle and invite in the elements and watchtowers, or whatever else inspires you. Follow the instructions for grounding and shielding in the beginning of this book.

Now is also the time to invite any deities, whether it's Aphrodite to awaken lust, longing, and Eros, or Shiva to connect with universal consciousness. If you are working partnered or with a group, I recommend inviting in no more than two deities, being sure that they complement one another. Use whatever language you like, formulating your intention and asking for their guidance, support, and compassion.

You also may wish to call in your highest erotic self, your Divine and sacred sexuality, or your fullest power. You may use an adapted version of the invocation in the last chapter, rewriting as you see fit:

> *I call upon my higher sexual self, my sacred sexuality, my erotic truth, to guide me in this ritual of activating and calling forth my fullest sexual expression and erotic power. May I be guided by forces and energies that work in my highest favor, in 100 percent light, so I may stand firmly in myself, as I am meant to. And so it is.*

Step 5: Mirror work or eye-gazing

If you are working with a partner, gaze into one another's left eyes (or right eye, just choose one). If an odd number of people are doing the ritual, someone may volunteer to eye-gaze twice or work with a mirror. If you are doing this ritual by yourself, gaze at your nondominant eye in the mirror.

The point of this part of the work is to dissolve all preconceived ideas of sexual and erotic power to make way for a new form of relating to the sensual self. You may repeat your affirmation or word of power out loud as you eye-gaze, but if you feel this is distracting you from being present, don't worry about it.

Begin by gazing into the eyes of your partner or your own in the mirror. Take a few deep breaths, and allow any worries, anxieties, or tension to leave with each exhale. Continue to hold your gaze and allow all insecurities and preconceived notions to melt away. You may see the face of your beloved or self melt away, rearrange, or open. Breathe into this. There's no pressure here for anything to happen. All you want is to allow presence, to fall into yourself and your power.

Once you feel yourself dropping into your body, into your power, into the moment, declare your intention out loud.

Step 6: Declaration of intention
As you gaze in the mirror or in the eye of a lover, state your intention. You may read or adapt the following or say whatever is in your heart; allow the moment to be the guide:

On this [the date] *day, with the Moon in* _____ *and the Sun in* _____, *I declare to the universe, to all witnessing guides* [and partners], *and to my higher erotic self, that I am ready to awaken the Divine Erotic within me and step fully into my sexual power. I declare that I am ready to claim my sensual potential and live up to it in all ways, always. So it is that I activate my intention,* [read your intention out loud], *so the universe may work with me and through me in making this my new reality. This or something better for the highest good of all involved. So mote it be!*

Take another moment to gaze in the mirror or in the eye of your lover. Feel the profundity of this declaration. Once you feel grounded, have each partner say their declaration out loud, repeating the process of holding space through breath and eye-gazing.

Step 7: Sex magick and circulation of energy

Now begin having sex or masturbating. You may reconnect with your affirmation or word of power, breathing in as you repeat it, and exhaling as you allow it to move through you. Allow this sex to be present, start slow, and try to circulate the energy as you practiced in the meditation on page 116.

For solo practice. As you feel the sexual energy moving through you, breathe it from your genitals to the crown of your head, and feel it pouring down your spine like a fountain, collecting at your genitals, creating a loop. Circulate the energy in this way, feeling it growing stronger and stronger with each pass, first up the spine and then down. As you feel the pleasure and sexual energy awaken, you may hold your word or affirmation in your mind's eye. Once you feel that it's getting to the point of no return, refocus on your intention. Feel the energy move from your genitals, up your body, through the crown of your head, and out into the universe, where it explodes into the cosmos and becomes reality. Spend time in the afterglow, feeling what it is like for your intention to manifest and to be grounded in your erotic potential.

For partnered practice. As you have sex, focus on your word or affirmation. You may wish to circulate the energy by creating a loop. As one of you inhales, the energy travels from the genitals, up to the heart, and through the mouth, where it connects with your lover's mouth; with the exhale, it moves through their mouth, down to their heart, and to their genitals. With your inhale, it passes back to you and into your heart. You can visualize creating this loop while in a position that doesn't allow kissing, too.

If there are more than two of you, focus on drawing the energy up from your genitals, through your heart, and through the crown of you head, where it pours forth like a fountain, moving back to your genitals and starting over. In other words, focus more on strengthening this energy within yourself. As you feel the energy rise, getting to the point of no return, focus on your intention once again, and feel the energy rising from the base of your spine to your heart, through the crown of your head. Feel it shooting into the cosmos, manifesting as your desire. If you didn't simultaneously orgasm, focus on supporting the intention of the partner who still needs to. Once everyone has orgasmed, or gotten as close as possible, spend time in the afterglow, feeling what it is like for your intention to manifest and to be grounded firmly in your sexual power.

Step 8: Create something to mark the boundary

You may write a new affirmation or work with the one you chose. You can create a piece of art, write a poem, invent a phrase that embodies your new relationship with the Divine Erotic, or even give yourself a new name to use during magick. Craft something that you can turn to that shows this transition or rite of passage. Allow your creativity to guide you. You may also pick a tarot card or archetype that embodies the way you want to step into your power, like the Lust/Strength card or the King of Wands.

Step 9: Close and ground

Perform the closing and grounding exercise from the beginning of this book. If you invited any deities into this ritual, thank them and let them know the working is done. Now is also the time to leave them offerings. You may also thank and dismiss your higher sexual self, adapting the following:

> *I thank my higher sexual self, my sensual soul, for guiding me in this ritual of activating and calling forth my fullest sexual expression and*

erotic power. This working is done, and the activation is complete. I thank you for your guidance. You may leave with peace. And so it is.

Perform the closing and grounding exercises. If you did the LBRP, now is the time to do a Qabalistic Cross. If you invited in the watchtowers and elements, now is the time to dismiss them. Basically, be sure to close whatever ritual you started. If you lit your sacred sex candle, snuff it out. You may wish to press your forehead into the ground like in child's pose, sending any excess energy into the earth. You may leave an offering of roses, chocolate, wine, mead, sweets, or whatever else resonates on your altar for your highest sexual self. Then go and give yourself an offering. Eat something delicious, take a bath, dance, or cry.

I also highly suggest taking this time to record what this ritual was like in your grimoire, noting whatever feelings, experiences, sensations, and visions came up. *And so it is.*

II

The Paths to
Sacred Sex

COSMIC GUIDANCE THROUGH
THE EROTIC JOURNEY

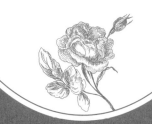

CHAPTER 4

Preparation for the Path

The path of the Divine Erotic begins in the flesh, although it expands to the subtle, to the layers of consciousness experienced in visionary and mystic states. The way to get there is intensely personal—not cookie-cutter but couture. Your path should be based on your own needs, experiences, and desires. And although you may have a conscious understanding of what sort of journey you want to pursue, you may not, and that's okay.

Because sex happens on the physical and energetic planes, it's important to work with tools that act in this same duo-focal way. We've already discussed erotic archetypes and tarot, and now let's really saunter in. My hope is that the paths of sacred sex to follow act as a starting point, not a destination, and that they help you carve out your own exploration of sacred sex that is totally and utterly personal.

PATHS OF SACRED SEX

In this section, you'll find the paths of Sacred Sex with their respective tarot archetypes and correspondences. Allow these to be a stepping stone onto the paths themselves, and take notice of what peaks your interest or resonates within you. Meditate and spend time with the card to dig deeper into its flavor of the Divine Erotic.

TEMPERANCE: THE PATH OF ALCHEMY

Hebrew letter and meaning: Samech, prop

Astrological correspondence: Sagittarius

Path on the Tree of Life: Tiferet (Beauty, the sphere of the Sun) to Yesod (Foundation, the sphere of the Moon)

Divinatory meaning: Finding balance between two opposing forces, the heart and will coming together in harmony, the need to purify and rectify to find a middle ground. Working with celestial and terrestrial forces to find a sense of balance and even-keeled movement forward.

About this path: This is the path of the erotic alchemist, who sees sex as a force of transformation, transmutation, and purification. This is a path of intense heat, of breaking down, of dissolution of the ego through the body as a way to become the most evolved version of yourself possible. This is spiritual alchemy through the use of sexual energy. This is the path of the Great Work of the flesh through the subversive, which uses traditions of spiritual alchemy alongside ritual to help you invoke your sexual power in a grounded and aligned way. This is the sexual alchemist's path through the balancing of the lunar and solar within.

THE LOVERS: THE PATH OF DIVINE UNION

Hebrew letter and meaning: Zayin, sword

Astrological correspondence: Gemini

Path on the Tree of Life: Binah (Understanding, the sphere of Saturn) to Tiferet (Beauty, the sphere of the Sun)

Divinatory meaning: The Divine Union of the solar and lunar, active and receptive aspects of self. A merging of the subconscious and conscious. A sense of love and romance with all life, or the new beginnings of love and relationship.

About this path: The Path of Divine Union utilizes relationship as a way to harness ecstasy and connection with the Divine, either through the beloved or through devotion to God/dess. This is the path of the sacred marriage, of devotion to other as a way to rectify duality within the self, the dance of merging with the energy of creation. This is the path of sacred relationship and conscious union, whether this is already in your life, or whether you want to call in this sort of relationship.

THE HIGH PRIESTESS: THE PATH OF THE MYSTIC

Hebrew letter and meaning: Gimel, camel

Astrological correspondence: The Moon

Path on the Tree of Life: Kether (the crown) to Tiferet (Beauty, the sphere of the Sun)

Divinatory meaning: A time of stillness and introspection. A sense of intuitive knowing and awareness through gnosis that can be harnessed by the subtle, by the esoteric, and by peeling back the veil of perception. A need to tune in to inner wisdom and mystical states of awareness for answers.

About this path: The path of the sacred slut and holy whore, this sees the erotic and sexuality as a way of honoring the Divine Feminine and the Divine Feminine within the self. This is the path of raising energy through sex as a method of transcendence and a way of aligning with the cosmic cycles. This is the path of the Goddess manifested through her aspect as Priestess of Love, who uses sexuality as a way of devotion and embodying cosmic consciousness. A path of embracing erotic intuition to guide you on your journey with sacred sex.

THE DEVIL: THE PATH OF THE DARK GOD/DESS

Hebrew letter and meaning: Ayin, eye

Astrological correspondence: Capricorn

Path on the Tree of Life: Tiferet (Beauty, the sphere of the Sun) to Hod (Splendor, the sphere of Mercury)

Divinatory meaning: The Devil speaks of a need to surrender to pleasure or to release addictions, bad habits, and moments of overindulgence. A reminder that you are the only one who's in control of your path and life, and that you are the only one who can liberate yourself from the chains of dogma. This can speak of going too far in the path of restriction or in the path of carnal pursuits. A message of one's own free will and God power.

About this path: This path explores subversive sexuality as a way to the Divine Erotic, through kink, BDSM, and altered states of consciousness. By working with the self as an embodiment and reflection of the Dark God/dess, this path utilizes taboos to break through self-imposed barriers. This is the Left Hand Path of intensity and transformation, through the practice of sacred sadomasochism, transgression, and self-worship.

THE EMPEROR:
THE PATH OF THE DIVINE EMBODIED MASCULINE

Hebrew letter and meaning: Heh, window
Astrological correspondence: Aries
Path on the Tree of Life: Chokmah (Wisdom) to Tiferet (Beauty, the sphere of the Sun)
Divinatory meaning: An omen of power that can be worked with and refined. The Emperor at its most evolved is the Divine Embodied Masculine; at his most encumbered state, he represents patriarchy and the abuse of power. This card represents the need to have a personal set of beliefs and ethics that allows you to share your resources wisely. It acts as a reminder of the activating and initiating power you have available to you at all times.
About this path: This is a path of rejecting internalized patriarchy and grounding in the powers of the Divine Masculine, of connecting with the unyielding potential in the self to impregnate the universe with Divine creation. Through the mysteries of the flesh and pleasure, the Emperor guides you in redefining masculinity in a way that embraces the feminine, as a means of achieving balance in the inner and outer worlds.

THE STAR: THE PATH OF EROTIC EMBODIMENT

Hebrew letter and meaning: Tzaddi, fishhook

Astrological correspondence: Aquarius

Path on the Tree of Life: Netzach (Victory, the sphere of Venus) to Yesod (Foundation, the sphere of the Moon)

Divinatory meaning: Divine guidance after a time of difficulty, connecting to one's purpose and path with clarity. A sense of being supported through a transition or process of evolution and transformation, and a renewed sense of faith and clarity at the path ahead. Being guided by your inner north star.

About this path: This is a path of embodiment and immanence that asks you to see the Divine in everything, especially the self. Filled with body worship and glamour, this approach centers the self and sexual self-expression as a way of aligning with the Divine Erotic. Through movement, adornment, and working with the body and the senses, you find the sacred sexual through rituals of self-lust and self-love.

SACRED SEX AS
SACRED EXPLORATION FOR . . .

Those paths outline few different ways to explore the Divine Erotic. They are the method of practice, one road your exploration may take, rooted in archetypal symbolism and personal significance. But the *reason* you want to begin on this journey will be unique. Whether you have survived sexual trauma and are ready to begin healing your relationship to sexuality, or you're ready for your own surrender to these erotic waters as an initiation into your fullest power, there is no wrong answer to why you're here.

In this section I offer a few reasons you may be starting on the path. Use the journal questions on pages 139–40 to untangle why you're here, and let these suggestions carry you forward with your erotic and esoteric exploits.

Self-love and self-lust: Your relationship with sacred sex may be a way of finding sexual liberation and empowerment through self-worship; through caring for the body and heart; and for finding joy and satisfaction for yourself physically, emotionally, and energetically.

Healing: If you are here to heal your relationship with sexuality, whether it's from sexual trauma, abuse, or simply living in a sex-negative and puritanical society, I just want to take a moment to witness your strength. The fact you are here in all your resilience is beautiful, and showing up is often the hardest step. You may wish to work through this book with a therapist, partner, or friend to support you on this journey.

Union: One of the goals of the Great Work is union of the higher and lower selves, or the rectification of the Divine and ever-living aspect of self that survives this incarnation, and the personality, ego, and self specific to this life and this body. This union of all aspects of the self can be honored, ritualized, and explored through working with sexual energy, the energy of life, magick, and the universe.

Initiation: One of the most meaningful and powerful aspects of my relationship with sacred sex is the way it has initiated me into my magick. When you commit to a life of sacred sex, the Divine Erotic infuses everything you bring your awareness to. Sex, met with awareness, has the ability to initiate you into new states of consciousness, new expressions of self, and new avenues of pleasure and power.

Pleasure: Pleasure is a guiding force. To deny this is to deny why humans love to eat, fuck, and lie in the sun—*it just feels good.* You may be exploring sacred sex as a foundation for physical pleasure or cosmic satisfaction. Sacred sex can be a bridge to both of these worlds and in moving from pleasure, which lies in the nervous system, to ecstasy, which transcends the self.

Conscious pain: Pain is part of the human experience, and it is also one of the oldest ways of exploring altered states of consciousness. From the Sun Dance of the Indigenous people of the American plains, to the self-flagellation of monks, to the hanging rites of the Brotherhood of the Flaming Arrow, pain is tied to spiritual rites. Pain in this context is the stream that leads into new avenues of the psyche and strength, into new avenues of sacred subversion, surrender, and sex.

Adventure: The world of sacred sex is one I hope you never stop exploring. Whether you are exploring solo or with others, this cosmic curiosity is everything. Even the most casual sex can have sacred implications when it's approached in an embodied way, grounded in the intention of adventure.

Your path will materialize in a way that resonates with *you*. You may know what this looks like already, or you may not. Use the following tarot spread to gain clarity around this and then use the sample paths to untangle how your own may manifest.

A TAROT SPREAD FOR FINDING YOUR PATH OF SACRED SEXUALITY

Use this spread to uncover where you can place your focus and then use the following examples of energetic paths to see what feels right and what doesn't. This doesn't mean your path will be exactly as the cards laid out. Rather, they will offer you a perspective into your subconscious needs or desires. Spend time journaling whatever it is you pull, meditating on the results, or creating art around it. As always, I invite you to turn your tarot pulls into a ritual. As you feel ready, shuffle the cards as you focus on your question, which may be specific or just, "What path of sacred sex is right for me?" Cut your deck if it's in your practice, pull your cards, and interpret. When you're done, record your results in your grimoire, taking the time to journal and explore.

Card 1: What's my inspiration for my path of sacred sex?
Card 2: Where in myself can I connect to this?
Card 3: How can I begin exploring this unique path?
Card 4: What do I need to keep in mind as I do so?
Card 5: What theme or message can I carry with me?

ORIENTING YOURSELF
ON THE PATH OF THE DIVINE EROTIC

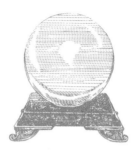

Sacred sex is many things, which can be overwhelming. When there's so much to do, feel, experience, touch, and explore, it can be difficult to figure out where to start. More than anything, a personal relationship with the Divine Erotic leads to *you*—the true you, unfiltered, stripped bare, lying on the altar of the body with limbs outstretched. To surrender means to expose the self, the whole self, and nothing but the self. But to get there means communing with your inner self, your higher sexual or erotic self, and the independent God/dess within you, the aspect of mutable Earth known as Virgo, the Virgin.

VIRGO, THE VIRGIN, AND THE HERMIT
AS THE ARCHETYPE OF EROTIC INDEPENDENCE

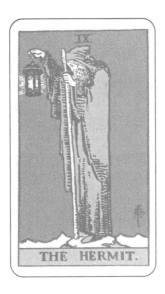

I won't lie to y'all. Virgo was one of those signs I just didn't get. My Aquarius and Scorpio self just never understood their energy and what I perceived as their refusal to be chill or chaotic in any way, shape, or form. I was seeing the exoteric nature of Virgo—the perfectionist, the type A personality, the person who always gets shit done and in the right way.

When I began studying the Virgin Goddess, this began to shift, and I was able to see the esoteric secrets of Virgo. The word *virgin*, to modern minds and interpretations, has been warped by patriarchy to mean someone inexperienced, a "prude," a sexuality that's defined by *lack*. But to the ancients of Sumer, Greece, Rome, and Egypt, virginity wasn't viewed in the same way. It was a mode of being that the Goddess embodied, not in a relation of lack to others, but one where sexuality was defined by being *whole unto one's self.* Virginity didn't mean anything but unmarried, and Artemis/Diana, Athena/Minerva, Hestia/Vesta, Asherah/Astarte, Inanna/Ishtar, Isis, and Aphrodite/Venus are all Virgin Goddesses. (Although Isis is married to Osiris, She is still considered a Virgin Goddess because Her relationship to Her sexuality is Her own.) Virginity was a relationship to the self, and that is the esoteric meaning of what Virgo can teach you.

The archetype of this grounded and malleable energy can teach you the way the body can bend to devotion while aligned with personal truth. The secret of Virgo is that it is a sexual sign in a way that honors the self above all. This power may be manifested through work and whatever is inspiring the person at that moment. Orienting yourself on the path of sacred sex as the virgin is vital. This means finding your own source of erotic inspiration, your own perspective, your own *intention.*

You can view the energy through the lens of its major arcana tarot card, the Hermit. The Hermit is the crone, the wise wo/man, the one who abandons all else to be in sacred communion with the self. All of Virgo's associations point back to the sacred center that lives in everyone and everything, the portal of the heart that allows you to access the secrets of the universe. The Hermit seeks union through solitude and represents this merging of the self with the Divine. Like the mystic poets of the Sufis, like the Song of Solomon in the Bible, like the Christian mystics, this union and merging is often described in erotic terms.

JOURNAL QUESTIONS

Allow the following questions to guide you to distinct possibilities within yourself. This chapter is more theoretical than the others, which means that journaling will help you break down and see how these concepts are within you and already manifested in your life. I invite you to answer whatever questions resonate as a jumping-off point.

Turn this into as much of a ritual as you'd like, using the tarot spread that follows to delve into your writing practice. Remember, wherever you are right here, right now, is absolutely perfect.

- What path of sacred sex do I feel *most* naturally drawn to? What is my intention in exploring this?
- What path of sacred sex do I feel *least* drawn to? Can exploring this path bring me a new perspective and sense of inner balance?
- What tarot card and archetype do I feel guiding me in this journey? What does this card/these cards activate within me?
- What are ways I can work with and embody this archetypal power?
- What sort of exploration does sex invite me into? How does this manifest in my life and spiritual practice?
- How does my relationship with my erotic self manifest energetically? What are practices I can work with to dive deeper into figuring this out?
- How does reframing my conception of virginity help me ground into my sexuality?

- How can the archetype of Virgo orient my relationship with sacred sex as something divine and personal *to me*?
- What are practices of self-care, self-love, and self-compassion that I can lean into as I begin my erotic explorations?

A TAROT SPREAD FOR SELF-CARE ON THE PATHS OF SACRED SEX

Use this spread to discover new ways to take care of yourself on this path, making sure to tend to your emotional, mental, physical, and spiritual body. If you wish, you may just use the twenty-two major arcana cards for this reading, working with their archetypal symbols and messages to better relate to the paths in the following chapters. You also are welcome to work with an oracle deck.

I invite you to turn this into a ritual, setting up the space as necessary, as laid out in Chapter 1. Focus on your question, whether it's about a specific path or something more general like, "How can I take care of myself as I walk the path of the Divine Erotic?" Shuffle the cards, cut the deck when you feel ready, and pull your cards of choice. Record your pulls and interpretations in your grimoire, and enjoy the clarity the cards bring you.

Card 1: What is the archetypal influence I am meant to connect to and work with?
Card 2: How can I ground and care for myself physically?
Card 3: How can I care for myself emotionally?
Card 4: How can I incorporate pleasure into my self-care routine?
Card 5: How am I supported in this journey?

AFFIRMATIONS

Once again, affirmations are here to help you incorporate the themes in this chapter into your daily life. These are here to help you remember the power you have on whatever path of sacred sexuality you choose. See them as a rainbow bridge to your essence, as muses and guides that can hold space as you transform through the radiant energy of sexual truth. Know that you can return to them whenever you need, no matter where you are in your journey, and use the steps in Chapter 1 to make the most of this practice.

- I prepare my mind, body, spirit, and soul for the path of sacred sex.
- I surrender to the power of the Divine Erotic.
- I embody the archetypal power of sexuality and allow this to guide me.
- I explore myself and my erotic energy with confidence and ease.
- I heal my relationship with sexuality by honoring all parts of myself.
- I go at my own pace and honor where I am right here, right now.
- I am exactly where I am meant to be.
- I am devoted to walking my personal path of Divine sexuality.
- I center myself in all ways and in all planes each time I begin exploring the path of the Divine Erotic.

- My sexuality and eroticism belong to no one but me, and I manifest this however I see fit.
- Through sacred sex, I open the door to vast possibilities of exploration.
- I allow the practice of sacred sex to expand all my perceptions of myself, my life, and magick.
- I care for myself with pride and gratitude in whatever ways I need, so I can remain centered in myself and my power.

A RITUAL CLEANSING BATH FOR BEFORE OR AFTER SACRED SEX

Your energy is a precious resource. Caring for this aspect of self is one of the most important foundational practices in any esoteric, occult, or magickal tradition; the same is true, and especially true, for sacred sex. Sex is as much an energetic act as a physical one. Sex pulls at the layers of body and soul to reveal something unknown and numinous. It requires radical vulnerability and trust in the self and others. Sacred sex is the erotic entanglement of the etheric and physical bodies. To show up fully to sacred sex means being aligned with and grounded in the energy body, and it means taking care of yourself spiritually. Ensuring everyone is cleansed and aligned with the Divine light/the cosmos/the universe/their higher sexual self is vital. If one of you brings your anxiety about work into the sacred space without cleansing, releasing, and grounding, don't be shocked if the other partner picks up on that energy. Sex is a conduit for transformation, so when you're plugged into someone's system, you will pick up on what they are experiencing.

I advise you do the grounding and shielding exercises that precede all rituals in this book as often as you can. Orienting yourself with the earth and heavens and protecting yourself through shielding is an integral practice, and the more you do it, the stronger the effects become. But this is just one way of caring for the etheric body. There are many others, including working with affirmations, visualization, taking spiritual baths, working with crystals, and practicing energy healing. Next, I will share a simple bath ritual (which can be adapted for a shower if you don't have a bath) that you can work with before and/or after you practice sacred sex, whether that's with a partner or partners or alone.

This ritual can be used before or after sacred sex, or whenever you feel like your etheric body needs a good cleanse. During the waning Moon is an optimal time to work with this practice, but don't let the lunar cycle limit you. Repeat this whenever you need to. You will be working with each element in this ritual. Your intention correlates to fire, the water to water, breath work and affirmation to air, and the herbs to earth. You—your spirit, your Divine Erotic essence—are the spirit that weaves it all together.

What you need: Epsom or pink Himalayan salt; a few pinches of herbs like thyme, nettle, rosemary, sage, peppermint, cascarilla (powdered egg shells), benzoin, juniper, mullein, or eucalyptus (try picking at least three herbs, which all have properties of protection, removing negative energy or curses, and cleansing the auric body; you can also use a couple drops of essential oil); a bath or shower (if you're using a shower, grab a canning jar and tea strainer or a French press to make an infusion); and some water to drink, especially if you like your baths hot.

Optional: A tea ball strainer or sachet, white candles, an oil diffuser, mood lighting, crystals you want to work with (just don't take porous crystals like selenite into the bath), and ambient music or tones playing. For after the bath, lotion, a dry brush, and massage oil.

You can practice this ritual with a partner if space permits. You may wish to share an intention and affirmation and practice in unison, or hold your individual intentions in your mind. You can also perform it separately but at the same time if you have two or more bathrooms.

Look over this ritual, *especially the breath work section*, before you begin.

Step 1: Set the space, and gather your supplies

If you have a bath, decide if you want to put the herbs straight into the tub or in a strainer to basically turn your bath into a tea. If you don't have a bathtub, you will pour the infusion over yourself in the shower as you follow the same ritual process.

Set the space. Draw your bath. If you are making an infusion, allow it to sit for at least thirty minutes ahead of time, if not longer (ideally, it would brew for twelve to twenty-four hours): put the loose herbs in the canning jar or French press, add boiling water, cover, and allow it to steep.

If you are taking this bath or shower before a sacred sex practice, you may take some time to tap into your sexuality through journaling, meditation, pulling tarot cards, dry brushing, or self-massage. You can also dance, practice yoga, or spend time outside. If you are doing it after your sacred sex practice, I invite you to see this as closing the ceremony as well as aftercare. Allow the ritual to help you integrate into normal, waking life.

Step 2: Pick your affirmation, and set your intention
Once the bath is set and the vibe is right, set your intention and pick an affirmation to anchor you to this intention. In this way, your affirmation helps you connect to the intention as you repeat your words of power. You may pull tarot or oracle cards to gain clarity, or journal and flip through this book for inspiration. While the point of this bath is to cleanse you and release stuck energy, there may be something specific you want to release, and that's where the intention and affirmation come in.

Intention: To cleanse my etheric, physical, astral, mental, emotional, and spiritual body of all negative energies, all impurities, and all blockages that are stopping me from aligning with 100 percent Divine light.

Affirmation: I cleanse and clear myself of all negative energies and impurities, on all planes and in all ways.

Intention: To cleanse and release tension, anxiety, worry, and blocks that are stopping me from being present and grounded in my erotic and sexual self. To release anything stopping me from pure presence and energy.

Affirmation: I cleanse and clear myself of all unnecessary energies, and I align myself with the pure possibility of presence.

Intention: To balance my energetic body, to release the energies I've picked up from others, to ensure I am healthy in spirit and energy so I may be centered while exploring the Divine Erotic.

Affirmation: I am balanced in all bodies, in all ways, and I am in perfect health energetically, erotically, and physically, always.

Write down your intention and affirmation in your Sacred Sex Grimoire, alongside what herbs you're using, what sign the Sun is in, what sign and phase the Moon is in, and what sort of sacred sex you're practicing before or after your bath.

Step 3: Add the salt and herbs, step into the bath or shower, and infuse it with energy

Before you step into the bath, add the salt and herbs or the tea infuser with the herbs that have been steeping. If you are taking a shower, run the water and be sure you have your infusion somewhere close by so you can grab it and check that it's not too hot. You will be pouring this over your body, so add cold water if it's too warm.

As you step in to the water, feel yourself as an embodiment of the eroticism of the cosmos. See yourself as Aphrodite or Eros or Poseidon or Oshun. Feel yourself and your body come in contact with the water. Feel the edges of the bath or the shower as it hits and kisses your skin. Allow the sensations to seduce and inspire you.

As you submerge yourself, come back to your affirmation. Allow the water to begin infusing it into you. As you feel ready, bless the bath or shower with energy. If you are in the bath, hold your palms parallel to the surface of the water. If you are in the shower, hold your palms parallel to the showerhead. Take a few deep breaths, and feel golden light ascending from the heavens into the crown of your head, down your spinal column, through your body and arms, and out your palms. Feel this golden light moving into the water and infusing it with purifying energy. If you practice reiki or other energy healing, give the bath some of this. Visualize the water turning golden or white, neutralizing any negative energy or impurities it may absorb from you through the power of the cosmos. Take a second to declare that this bath or shower is sanctified in the name of the Divine Erotic and that it is a healing portal to bask in.

Step 4: Declare your intention out loud

Once you feel your bath or shower water is blessed, declare your intention. You may say something like the following, or speak from the heart. You will be using your affirmation to solidify your intention out loud while holding your palms parallel to the water.

> I declare this bath/shower is sanctified in the name of the Divine Erotic and that it is a portal to purification and healing that works on all planes. I am cleansed, cleared, and balanced of all negativity. [State your affirmation.] And so it is.

Step 5: Purify yourself

Purify yourself by dunking your head under the water if you're in the bath or by pouring your infusion over your head and body if you're in the shower. Feel yourself letting go and releasing all that's not aligned with your most erotic, divine, sexual self. Each time you dunk your head, feel yourself being baptized by the Divine Erotic and cleansed of anything that doesn't serve your highest sexual self. If you are pouring your infusion over your head, feel this as a waterfall of purification, washing over you and releasing anything you no longer need as it moves down the drain.

Step 6: Practice breath work and then soak

Breath work will align you with the elemental energy of earth (the square breath), to ground, or with water (the triangle breath), to further cleanse your spiritual body.

> *Earth breath:* To ground, to be more present in the body, to find balance between all aspects of yourself.
> *To practice:* Inhale . . . hold . . . exhale . . . hold. Then repeat.
> *Water breath:* To purify, to sink deeper into your emotional body, to clear and release any stuck emotions or feelings.
> *To practice:* Inhale . . . exhale . . . hold. Then repeat.

Pick your breath of choice, starting with four seconds for each part and then adding time as you feel comfortable. Repeat for a few minutes or as long as you'd like. Breath work is meant to be a challenge but not a struggle. Go at your own pace. You may repeat a shortened version of your affirmation for each part of the breath as well.

Once you feel balanced, soak in the tub or enjoy your shower, repeating your intention or affirmation as you do. Water carries vibrations, has a memory, and will absorb and hold your intention, transmuting it into Divine light thanks to the charging you did. Allow the water to nourish you, and feel it absorbing or washing away any energetic impurities, any negative energy, anything others have thrust on you without your consent. Stay here for as long as you'd like.

Step 7: Drain the water

Once you feel that the water has absorbed all the energy it can, and when you feel balanced and purified, pull the tub stopper or turn off the shower. If you are draining the tub, stay in the water as it drains. Feel the way it grazes at the edge of your skin as it gets more and more shallow. Anything negative is getting flushed down the drain, back into the earth, where it will be transmuted and cleared.

Step 8: Close the purification

Step out of the tub. Repeat your affirmation to yourself. Thank yourself, the water, and the herbs for their support and healing. Allow yourself to be nourished and held by this ritual. And so it is.

Don't forget to drink water! If you are going on to perform sex magick, you may adorn yourself, working with glamour to step into the most magickal version of yourself possible. If you are using this rite to finish a sacred sex working, you may now eat some food and go about the rest of your day.

If you put herbs straight into the tub, allow them to dry before removing them for easier cleanup.

OTHER WAYS TO CLEANSE YOURSELF BEFORE OR AFTER SACRED SEX

There are numerous ways to care for your psychic, spiritual, and energetic health to ensure you're as aligned as possible before engaging in sacred sex. Here are some ideas:

- Use a selenite wand to sweep your body, visualizing it neutralizing any negative energy.
- Meditate with black crystals like onyx, obsidian, or black labradorite. Feel them absorbing any energy that is not aligned with 100 percent Divine light, with the cosmos, or with your higher sexual self.
- Practice banishing and healing rituals like the Lesser Banishing Ritual of the Pentagram or the Middle Pillar ritual.
- Practice grounding and shielding meditations.
- Work with affirmations that declare yourself and your energy sovereign, uninfluenced, and unaffected by negative energy.
- Visualize yourself under a waterfall of white light that cleanses and purifies you of negative, unneeded energy.
- Dance and move your body as you feel the physicality of this releasing and banishing any negative energy.
- Practice breath work with the earth or water breath to ground and clear your body.
- Cleanse yourself with sacred smoke as you feel and visualize all energy that is not yours and that does not vibrate in 100 percent Divine light leaving your etheric and erotic being.

RITUALS FOR ENERGETIC SEXUAL HYGIENE AND PSYCHIC PROTECTION

After a good ol' fashioned romp in bed, nothing hits the spot quite like a shower. Even the quickest of bathing rituals is a powerful refresh in and of itself. This is true both on a physical level and an energetic or spiritual level, like when you're washing less-than-stellar sex. Just as you use condoms or take birth control and have the STI conversation with potential boos, so does the sex witch too take into consideration the energetic implications of sex.

As you explore the paths of sacred sex, whether alone or with a partner, you want to make sure that you're taking care of your soul and spirit as much as your body. With sex comes engaging with someone's energy in the most intimate way possible. To make sure that you're not picking up on any of their unresolved issues, anxieties, doubts, or insecurities, take matters into your own hands by cleansing yourself before and after sex. This is a way of maintaining your boundaries, your spiritual hygiene, and your mental balance. Though it may not be necessary every time you have sex, especially if you're in a committed relationship or relationships, it can be useful, especially with sex magick dynamics, during casual sex, and during the dating process when you're still getting to know someone.

Here are some simple rituals that you can work with before or after sex to protect yourself and align with the energy of the cosmos.

Align with the Divine light. One of my favorite visualizations is one in which you align your being with Divine, healing light from each direction. This can be done before or after sex or as a daily practice outside of any sexual context at all. After finding a comfortable seat, close your eyes, and come back to your breath. As you begin to feel a sense of peace and space, visualize the heavens above as brilliant white light pouring through you, moving through the crown of your head, down your spine, and piercing into the earth, so you are immersed in and one with this pillar of healing energy. Then visualize this same healing energy on your right hand, moving through your right shoulder, through your heart, and out your left shoulder. This pillar of light is infinite, with no beginning or end. Feel this energy from above and below and from side to side, overlapping at your heart. Then see this same white healing energy before you, moving through your chest, through your heart, and out the back of your body, extending infinitely before you and behind you. Now you have three pillars of light: above and below, side to side, and back to front. Breathe into your heart space where the light overlaps and then into your whole body and being until you are glowing, radiating, and basking in this light from each direction. The light from your heart grows and grows until you are nothing but infinite light, held together by the potential of the universe. Stay here as long as you need.

You can also practice this visualization with different colors and energies. If you want to channel the kinky fire of Mars, you could visualize red light moving through you in each direction. If you want to work with the communicative and magick of Mercury, you can work with orange light.

Bloom like a rose. Find a comfortable position in which to meditate, taking deep breaths until you're present. Feel a radiant gold light spreading from all directions, into and through your heart, and growing and moving throughout your body. Bask in this golden veil of love and protection. Then, as you're ready, tap into your heart. As you inhale, visualize your heart as a giant blooming rose, each of its petals unfurling. As you exhale, the petals close just a little, but the flower still remains open. As you breathe in again, the rose blooms more and more, and as you exhale, it flutters in the wind. Repeat this until you feel centered, open, and loving.

This rose can be any color you want, or you can try white or gold for protection, red for passion, or pink for romance.

Shower in protective light. Find a safe space for meditation and get into a comfortable position. Pay attention to your breath, and anchor into the present moment. Visualize the heavens above as striking white light, the source of all protection and healing. Then feel this light pouring down like a waterfall or rain, and the healing white energy washing away any energetic impurities, any worries, anything that's stopping you from being your most vibrant, centered, and magickal self. Stay in this cleansing, healing light as long as you need.

Different colors align with different frequencies and qualities that you want to bring into the bedroom, or as a way to balance whatever happened during sex. So if you had kinky sex and want to feel nourished and cared for, you may visualize blue or golden light for healing. If you want to feel romantic and loving, you can feel yourself being washed over with Venusian colors like pink or green.

Practice shielding with your partner. In this visualization, you will protect your own energy while also creating a safe container for your lover. Like in the basic shielding you've learned, begin in meditation, by drawing light down from the heavens and up from the earth. Practice extending this out from your heart to create a sphere of protection—except in this instance your two individual spheres of protection will merge into one. Meditate next to or in front of one another, pulling in energy from above and below, breathing and seeing your individual spheres of protection, and then seeing the spheres coming together. You can pick a color to help channel a specific energy into the sex you'll have as well. After, visualize the sphere you've connected separating back into your individual spheres of protection. Each of you will breathe this back into your heart spaces, where it dissolves, following the normal closing routine for shielding.

This is a powerful ritual to do before sex magick because it helps to hold the energy until you're ready to send it out into the universe. It can also protect you from any lingering energies or spirits that may have been attracted to the energy you've raised.

Cut the cord. Sometimes you simply need to disconnect from someone else's energy. Maybe the relationship is imbalanced, not reciprocal, or disrespectful. Sometimes the vibe is just off and you need a fresh start. Cord cutting is a way of energetically releasing connections (aka etheric or energetic cords) you unconsciously create with others, including those you have sex with. These cords are energetic attachments that come from relating to someone, thinking of how they perceive you, thinking of how they perceive you perceiving them, and so on—a domino effect of energy. They happen with anyone you interact with, and with sex, these cords are strengthened. To practice cord cutting, find your way to meditation. Find a comfortable position, and ground and shield. Then visualize yourself bathing in a violet flame that begins to dissolve all the cords that you no longer need. You may feel your connection to the specific person you want to cut cords with. You can call upon Archangel Michael, archangel of protection with the flaming sword, to help you cut the cord. Feel this beam of energy connecting you to this other person. Know that cord cutting releases your energetic ties but doesn't banish them. This is a practice in releasing, and if the relationship is meant to continue, it will in a new way. Ask Archangel Michael to assist you in cutting this cord, feeling his flaming sword slicing through the connection, healing the pain in you, and allowing you freedom to move forward, whole unto yourself. Stay here as long as you need, until you feel the cord dissolved into golden light. Thank Michael and then practice the finishing grounding and shielding exercises.

CHAPTER 5

The Path of Alchemy

A spiritual life, a magickal life, a mystical life full of sex and spirit is one of radical vulnerability, surrender, and fortification. To commit yourself to awakening often means facing the darkest corners of the self with bravery, even when it feels like you're transforming in a way that is gut-wrenchingly painful. This is the Great Work, one of shedding and releasing, of purifying, of aligning the macrocosmic and microcosmic, of finding the truth of the universe through the flesh.

This is the path of alchemy. The alchemical path can look like many things, and in this case, it will revolve around the spiritual, sexual, and energetic transformation that takes place when one dances with the Divine Erotic. Alchemy is the art of transmutation, or of transforming one substance into another of a more refined grade or higher quality—classically of a base metal into a silver or gold. One can work through the process of spiritual or inner alchemy, too, as a method of purification and evolution of the soul. And *that* is what we're talking about. Erotic alchemy views the body as the beaker, the soul as the substance to be transmuted, and the conscious energetic awareness of the sexual self as the change agent.

Alchemy is a process of breaking down a substance into its separate parts, purifying these parts, rejoining them, and then purifying them again to build something that's stronger than it was originally. The spiritual or erotic alchemist turns their gaze inward and uses the tools of spirituality and sexuality to accomplish this same work through visualization, meditation, ritual, movement, prayer, invocation, introspection, and total honesty, not to mention sex.

When you commit to the path of transformation alone, this work is hard enough. But when you walk alongside someone else in a sacred relationship, this becomes even more difficult, as your own shit is mirrored and reflected in their awakening. No matter what you choose, this is not an easy journey because a big part of the alchemical process is burning away what makes the foundation of the self—the patterns, the rigidity, the complexes. These are sacrificed to the alchemical furnace through the powers of the erotic, where they are transfigured and offered up to the beloved, the Divine, or the cosmos. This is calcination, where the base material is reduced to ash.

This commitment, if you take it up, is one that will revolutionize your world. And it's not the world itself that changes, but *you*. And that changes everything.

THE ALCHEMY OF SEX

While there is alchemy in the laboratory, in the physical vessels and the literal transmutation of substances, emotional or spiritual alchemy illustrates the power of attention, energy, and devotion to radically change oneself. The Path of Alchemy in sacred sex lends this same lens to the erotic, as all triggers and happenings in one's sexual life act as a catalyst for deep transformation. This means that the pain, the darkness, the depths of one's own shadows around lust and sexuality, no matter how painful they are, can act as triggers for soul-level evolution.

The Philosopher's Stone, which is the goal of alchemical work and is made from the transmutation of a base metal into gold, represents the "holiness of divine opposites." According to Paracelsus, the Philosopher's Stone is constructed through "union and transformation of Sulphur and salt, compared to the union of sol and Luna"; this can be thought of as the duality and polarity within each person that the alchemical process aims to unite. To the Taoist, this is represented as yin and yang; in Jungian terms, it's the unconscious and conscious; and in Kabbalistic terms, it is the union of Shekinah (or the Feminine Divine) and the Godhead. This act of merging is the alchemical marriage, and the result is the birth of a new soul and body. This is seen in the Lovers tarot card, in the hexagram with the upward and downward triangles of ascent and descent coming together. The alchemical process is also seen in the Temperance tarot card, which is the guiding archetypal force for this path.

The spiritual alchemist works on one's own soul, and sex and eroticism act as a gateway to this that's untouched by anything else. Because sex raises energy, and because it is such a vulnerable and intimate act, the potential for true transformation here is potent. Alchemy is the process of merging opposites, and this literally takes place during sex when two bodies come together, or when the self becomes the lover and finds the bridge between its own polarities, known as the sacred or alchemical marriage. Crowley described the alchemical marriage as "an ecstatic surrender to one's inner self"—even the conjoining of two people could be seen as the beloved reflecting one's inner or Divine nature to the self. The sex magician utilizes flesh, blood, and self as the alchemical laboratory and works with orgasms and erotic energy as the potent tools of transformation and bridge to the Great Work. When soul (sulfur), spirit (Mercury), and body (salt) come into harmony, an energy of ecstatic union occurs. This could be thought of as living the Divine Erotic.

TEMPERANCE AND THE PATH OF SAMECH

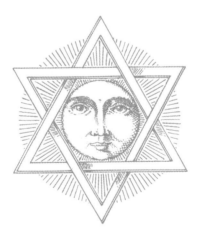

The archetypal example of the Alchemical Path of the Divine Erotic is Temperance, one of the two alchemical cards of the Tarot, alongside that of the Lovers, Gemini's card, which sits across the zodiacal axis from Sagittarius, the sign attributed to Temperance. These two cards are complements, and as you explore the Path of Divine Union, you will see how they each play a role in exploring Eros. Whereas the Lovers focus on union, Temperance shows the esoteric secrets of what makes this possible, allowing one to pass through the veil to the hidden laboratory within, where Sol and Luna are ready and waiting to reveal their secrets.

Temperance works with the heat of sexual energy to transform something from a lower vibration to a higher one. In the classic Smith-Waite deck, you see the archangel Michael with a chalice in each hand, pouring water from cup to cup. Michael pours the waters of the unconscious from chalice to chalice, representing transformation through bringing loving awareness and attention to intensity and darkness. He represents what's necessary to commit to before one can pass into other realms of existence; to experience or be truly embodied in the Divine Union with the beloved, the self must be grounded in the soul and body, which can only come after the alchemical preparations have been done. In the Thoth tarot deck, the Temperance card is called "Art" and is depicted as fire becoming water and water becoming fire.

Temperance speaks of balance and surrender, of moving through the portal of the heart by way of the subconscious, as it connects the spheres of the Sun (Tiferet/Beauty) and the Moon (Yesod/Foundation) on the Tree of Life. This balance of polarity is seen in Vajrayana Buddhism in the Red and White drops, in tantra as Shakti and Shiva, in Taoism as the yin and the yang, in gnostic Christianity as Jesus and Mary, and in Hermeticism as the triangles that encompass the hexagram. Temperance moves through the Middle Pillar on the Tree of Life, which reflects this same balance between force and form, active and receptive, feminine and masculine.

But there's also a sexual secret to this card that speaks of a physical merging of dualities. The solar sphere of Tiferet (Beauty) is the sixth sphere on the Tree, and the lunar sphere of Yesod (Foundation) is the ninth, which makes their link through Temperance the Path of 69. What's more, this is the alchemical union of Sol and Luna, or the polarities of solar and lunar between two individuals (regardless of gender because everyone has all energies within them) finding balance by dissolving into one another. This is reflected in Michael pouring from cup to cup, which could be thought of as "the elixir" or the sacred mixture of sexual secretions. This is symbolized both by the act of mutual oral sex, or 69, and by the conjunction of forces symbolized through consummation, or the ritual of Hieros Gamos or sacred marriage. (Originally, the sacred marriage was an erotic ritual of fertility that represented the cycles of birth, sex, death, and rebirth that reflected the renewal of the crops. Eventually, it was turned into a ritual during which a High Priestess embodying the Goddess would have ritualized sex with a King to pass on his ability to carry the throne.)

The following ritual works with sexual secretions, which are especially potent in combination, the merging of Sol and Luna, and the option of 69ing as a way to invoke the potencies represented by the Temperance card.

WAYS TO WALK THE ALCHEMICAL PATH

Part of this work is knowing when to surrender. Knowing when to stay in the furnace, in the heat, for a bit longer. Knowing when the time comes to hermetically seal yourself and go within, observing the erotic self being born. Sexuality ebbs and flows, and sometimes that means the sexual current is turned inward and needs time before it's naturally drawn out exoterically. The integration process is crucial, and this could mean celibacy or taking time as a single human when you're in a relationship. Or, after long periods of engaging solo with the Divine Erotic within the self, you may naturally yearn to share it with others.

These suggestions are meant to help you take this practice throughout your life, no matter where you are on your journey. There is no end to the work. Every relationship, every experience, every hookup is an opportunity to evolve.

IF YOU ARE IN A RELATIONSHIP OR MULTIPLE RELATIONSHIPS

- Engage in sex (whatever that means *to you*) as a way of diving into the problems and issues you're facing. See the coming (or cuming) together of bodies as the alchemical furnace, and allow the heat of making love to sublimate whatever you're tossing into the fire.

- Honor disagreements, projections, jealousy, and the rising of the shadow self as an invitation to go further into whatever is bringing them up. *Engage with* the difficult stuff, not trying to reject it or shut it down to make things easier. An open heart and honest communication are everything.

- Honor your relationship(s) as the container for evolution, both as individuals and as the way you commit to grow together, so you can weave a synastry that's complemented by your individual dedication to the work.

- Devote time individually and as a couple or couples to unravel how the Divine Erotic shows up in your life and what sacred sex means to you both.

- See your own relationship to sexuality as a means to showing up more thoroughly in an erotic alchemical relationship. Use personal taboos and your erotic edge to help you get here.

- Remember that just as there are many stages in the alchemical process, so is true of your union(s). Everyone has the chance to evolve into a container for the awareness necessary to move into a higher state of being and consciousness.

IF YOU'RE SINGLE

- See lovers and relationships as a path into the mysteries of the self by honoring any triggers, annoyances, jealousy, and problems as your alchemical ingredients. They're all fodder for alchemy if you look through the lens of radical acceptance.

- Engage with sex and masturbation as a form of devotion to your erotic energy. This means knowing that your sexuality isn't defined by anyone else, but rather is something that you get to share with others.

- Take periods of celibacy to focus your energy inward for self-exploration, feeding your own desires and honoring where you are.

- Honor sexual relationships of all kinds, whether casual or committed, as a means of self-mastery by welcoming in whatever issues, complexes, difficulties, or vulnerabilities come up rather than shying away from them.

- Converse with, explore, and know the shadow self in sex to guide you into a more integrated self. Honor limits, taboos, fears, complexes, desires, and boundaries and safely push up to your edge as a way to know yourself more completely.

- Work with your sexual fluids in spells and rituals, using them, for example, to anoint yourself or talismans, and seeing your body as the alchemical vessel.

JOURNAL QUESTIONS

The Path of Alchemy is a heady one, and as alchemy itself is a branch of magick with thousands of books written on the subject, it can be a deep dive. The following questions are here to help you break down what you read so you can take the alchemical process into your own exploration. Journaling helps you sort out how to incorporate the practices and philosophies that resonate in your own life.

You may wish to work with the following tarot spread before turning to the journal prompts. Set your space and answer whatever questions feel right, allowing them to lead you where you're meant to be. And so it is.

- How does approaching spiritual alchemy as a container for sacred sexuality deepen your connection to the Divine Erotic?

- How does seeing your relationships as a vessel for transformation allow you to embrace life and its range of experience?
- What does it mean to be an erotic alchemist? How can this understanding help you show up more fully in sex?
- What does it mean for you to walk the Path of Alchemy? How can you see the pain and joy and ecstasy of sex as a path to soul-level transformation?
- What do you hope to transform through erotic alchemy?
- What are the ways that you are hoping to grow along this path?
- How can working with sexual fluids become a part of your practice? How can you begin to release judgment around this taboo and instead see it as an offering of flesh and spirit?
- How does erotic alchemy help you find more presence, understanding, and connection with your sexual partners? How can it help you see bumps in the road as avenues to transformation?

A TAROT SPREAD
FOR WALKING THROUGH THE FIRE

Walking any path of the Divine Erotic has its challenges, and the Path of Alchemy especially so. It requires surrender to all experiences, as it's the coarse, dark material of the shadow that you are transmuting into consciousness. It can also feel isolating if you don't have people in your life who understand why you're consciously inviting in pain and vulnerability.

The following tarot spread, which also can be used with oracle cards, will act as a guide. Set up yourself and your space to feel embodied and magickal as fuck. Before you begin, think of the question you want to ask the cards. Shuffle the cards as you keep your question in mind. Split the deck if it's in your practice, pull the cards, and record the spread in your grimoire. Interpret them using your intuition as a guide, and come back to this spread whenever you need.

Card 1: Where can I allow the alchemical fire to burn away old habits, patterns, and fears around sex and the erotic?

Card 2: How can I surrender to this?

Card 3: How can I work with erotic alchemy to evolve my soul?

Card 4: How can I work with sacred sex to accomplish this?

Card 5: How can I stay grounded in my erotic essence through the intensity?

AFFIRMATIONS

Remembering your power *is vital* as you find your way into this underworld of the self. One way to do this is through affirmations, which by now, you are more than familiar with. Repeat these before or after sex magick, when you go through an alchemical working that feels especially potent, or when you need to remember who you are and where you're going. As always, these are an invitation to conceive your own; take the ones that strike a chord and leave the rest. Work with the steps laid out in Chapter 1 to make the most of your affirmations.

- I am an erotic alchemist.
- I walk the Path of Alchemy, step into the furnace, and come out transformed.
- Everything in my life offers me the chance to evolve and transform.
- My sexuality is a potent alchemical force.
- I transmute and transform through the potency of sacred sexuality.
- My sexuality is a force of nature.
- I honor the Divine Erotic as a path of evolution.
- My relationships and partners help me create a container for alchemical transformation.
- I surrender to the heat of erotic alchemy and allow it to move through me.
- My sexuality offers me a path of growth and soul-level expansion.
- I am grounded, empowered, and divinely guided on the path of erotic alchemy.
- I am in a constant state of sexual metamorphosis.
- I transcend my limitations and work with my erotic essence to do so.

LIBER 69: A SOLAR AND LUNAR INVOCATION AND RITUAL OF THE ALCHEMICAL MARRIAGE

This ritual is inspired by the esoteric secrets of Temperance, the alchemical merging of Sol and Luna, and the mixing of the sacred elixir that brings forth their currents. In this ritual, you and your partner will be aligning with the energies of Temperance and invoking one or both of the luminaries (the Sun and the Moon) before engaging in mutual oral sex or masturbation. The intention is to perform an erotic alchemical working by utilizing sexual energy to unite the solar and lunar selves, using sexual secretions to do so.

Before you begin: If you are performing this ritual with a partner, decide who will be invoking the Sun and who will be invoking the Moon. Allow whichever resonates with you more to dictate this. You also may look at your birth charts; whoever has more Cancer or fourth house influence may invoke Luna, and whoever has more Leo or fifth house influence may invoke Sol.

If you are performing this ritual solo, my suggestion is to invoke whichever luminary you feel *less* connected to. That way, you'll balance these energies within you.

This working is especially potent on a Sunday or Monday (these days are ruled by the Sun or the Moon, respectively), during a full Moon (when the light of the Sun is reflected on the Moon), when the Sun or the Moon is in Leo or Cancer (these signs are ruled by the Sun and the Moon, respectively), when the Sun or the Moon is in Sagittarius (this is the sign associated with Temperance) or on the equinoxes, or when day and night hang in equal balance. If it's a

Sunday, you may wish to perform the ritual at the hour of the Moon, and if it's a Monday, at the hour of the Sun. You can use an app or online planetary hour calculator to help determine this.

What you need: The Temperance, Sun, and High Priestess cards on your altar; a gold and a silver candle in candleholders; matches or a lighter; your grimoire; and incense like jasmine, vanilla, or ylang ylang for the Moon or amber or frankincense for the Sun.

A note: If you are doing this with a partner, make sure you have been tested for STDs and that you are fluid bonded. Being a responsible and ethical sex witch is of the utmost importance on any path of sacred sex.

And just one more note: There is an option for working with the Hebrew intonations of the spheres and energies you will be invoking. If you have no idea what I'm talking about, feel free to skip these steps.

Step 1: Set up the space and altar, and set your intention

By now you should be familiar with the steps it takes to build a sacred sex ritual. As always, start by preparing yourself and the space. You may perform a bath ritual (page 142) or spend time outside under the Sun or the Moon. You can purify yourself with sacred smoke, breath work, or movement. Adorn yourself in the metals that correspond to the luminary you will be invoking: Luna is silver and Sol is gold.

Gather your supplies. You may place the corresponding tarot cards on your altar: Temperance, the Sun for the Sun, and the High Priestess for the Moon (*not* the Moon card, confusingly). Cloak yourself in a robe that's gold or yellow, silver, or sheer, or you can work skyclad (naked) if you prefer.

Now set your intention with your partner, if you have one. While the purpose of this working is to balance the solar and lunar energies, and to work with erotic alchemy to rectify the dualities of these energies, you may have a more exoteric or specific intention as well. Maybe you feel as if there's an abundance of active solar energy in your relationship that is causing everything to feel combustible and explosive, and you need the tempering and intuitive energy of the Moon. Or maybe you feel as if your relationship with your sexuality is too internal, too mental, and that it's time to manifest this through a more embodied expression of eroticism that you are able to share with other people through Sol. Spend time journaling, using the questions and tarot spread in the previous sections, and then write your intention clearly. You may state it using the following formula:

I declare that by this working and by drawing down the energies of Sol and Luna, through the art of erotic alchemy, that [State your intention.].

Step 2: Ground and center
After you have your intention set and your temple space set up, ground and center using the instructions in Chapter 1.

Step 3: Call on the Path of Temperance, invoke Sol and Luna, draw down their energy, and light candles
Take a moment to move toward the altar. Stand before the Temperance card. Breathe into this card to feel what it says to you. Don't think of its associations or its esoteric meaning. Just gaze at the card as if it were your first time. When you feel ready, you may say the following out loud, solo or with your partner, or write something that resonates:

I/We stand now on the Path of Temperance, the Path of Samekh, that leads from Sol to Luna, the alchemical and divine union of the luminaries. I/We call forth this energy to move through me/us, to rectify duality through the current of sacred sexuality. May Temperance guide me/us in this ritual of erotic alchemy, for the highest good of all involved, and aligned with my/our True Will(s).

If it is in your practice, you may vibrate the letter Samekh, inhaling deeply and then intoning in a low voice:

SAHHHHH-MEEEEHHHHCCCCC.

Close your eyes and feel this declaration of the path moving through you.

Now you will be drawing down the light of whatever luminary you're invoking.

If you are invoking the Sun: Visualize its yellow-gold sphere above your head, and breathe as you draw this energy down through the crown of your head. Work slowly, feeling this activating, cleansing, and energizing golden light moving through each part of your body. By the time it gets to the tips of your toes, you are illuminated from the inside out.

If you are invoking the Moon: Visualize its silver sphere above your head, and breathe as you draw this energy down through the crown of your head. Work slowly, feeling this calming, restorative, mystical, and cooling silver light moving through each part of your body. By the time it gets to the tips of your toes, you are illuminated from the inside out.

When you, and your partner, feel filled with the light of the luminary you are invoking, you will light the candles. Each partner will light their respective candle. If you are doing this solo, you will light both.

Now invoke whichever planetary energy you are materializing, beginning with the Sun and then moving to the Moon (because the sphere of the Sun comes first on the Tree of Life).

If you are invoking Sol, say the following as you visualize yourself dissolving and reforming as the Sun. Or you may visualize it without a verbal declaration or speak from the heart instead:

Oh, Sol, embodied through Beauty, luminary of the heart and center of all, seat of wisdom and consciousness, I call upon you now and invoke your vitality and life-giving energy within me. I call forth your passion, your celestial activation, your golden grace and brightest expression so I may feel your radiance within me, in this alchemical erotic activation through the Path of Temperance.

If it is in your practice, vibrate the Divine Name of Tiferet, the Sun: Yod Heh Vav Heh Eloa Vada'at, inhaling deeply and then intoning in a low voice:

YOD HEH VAV HEH EL OH AH VA DAH AHHHTTTT.

If you are invoking the Moon, say the following as you visualize yourself dissolving and reforming as Luna. Or you may visualize it without a verbal declaration or speak from the heart instead:

Oh, Luna, embodied through the Foundation, luminary of intuitive wisdom and understanding, seat of the mysteries and subconscious, I call upon you now and invoke your shadowy power that cuts through all darkness into me at this time. I call forth your inner illumination, your stoic power of cooling and calming, your cyclical nature and psychic expression so I may feel your sanctity within me, in this alchemical erotic activation through the Path of Temperance.

If it is in your practice, vibrate the Divine Name of Yesod, the Moon: Shaddai El Chai, inhaling deeply and then intoning in a low voice:

SHAD EYEEEE EL HAIIIII.

Now close your eyes. Feel yourself as Sol or Luna, not analyzing what you feel or why, but simply noticing the what. Feel the energy from above moving through you, and know that the invocation is working, even if you don't feel a huge shift.

Step 4: Statement of intention and declaration

Declare the intention of your working. Stand before your altar and candles, and read what you wrote out loud, together with your partner if applicable, as you feel the energy moving through your body, through your lungs, out of your mouth, and know that you are bringing this declaration into reality.

Repeat your intention, using the following as inspiration:

I declare that by this working on the Path of Temperance, by drawing down the energies of Sol and Luna, through the art of erotic alchemy that [State your intention.].

When you're done, feel this energy coursing through you and out into the universe.

Step 5: Sex magick through 69ing and circulating energy

Now you will be embodying Sol and Luna by seeing your body as the Path of Temperance/Samekh that connects them. You will circulate Lunar and Solar energy throughout your body, whether you are doing this solo or partnered.

Get into position to 69 or to masturbate, and as you breathe, feel yourself as the luminary you invoked, drawing down its light into your body.

If you are partnered: While you 69, as you inhale, you draw forth the energy of the luminary you invoked, and as you exhale, you send this energy through your body and into your partner's body, creating a circuit of energy from the mouth to genitals. Don't get too caught up in thinking of what energy is going where—the working is *working*.

If you are solo: While you masturbate, feel yourself as the luminary you invoked, and draw down the energy of the other luminary into your body.

If you invoked Sol, inhale Lunar energy, and exhale as you feel it mixing with Solar energy. If you invoked Luna, breathe in Solar energy, and exhale as you feel it mixing with Lunar energy.

Whether you're partnered or solo, you may also visualize the astrological glyph for your luminary to cultivate this connection. *Stay here until you feel ready to move on.* You may feel your body begin to buzz, or you may feel yourself wrapped in light. Trust that even if you feel nothing, the magick is still happening.

Step 6: Send out the energy

If you are partnered: When you feel that you're going to orgasm, or that you and/or your partner are at the peak of your energy raising, hold the intention in your mind, and as you climax, send out energy through the crown of your head and through your genitals, so it goes into the cosmos and through the body of your partner. Even if you don't orgasm at the same time, keep your mouth on one another's genitals until the other partner orgasms or gets as close as possible, and have them repeat the process while both of you hold the intention in your mind. When you are both done, take whatever sexual fluids were produced in your mouths, and pass them to your partner by kissing. Feel yourselves as Sol and Luna embracing, becoming the chalices in the Temperance card. When you feel ready, split the fluid between your mouths and swallow, feeling your bodies charged with the nectar of the Sun and Moon.

If you are solo: As you feel yourself about to orgasm, or getting as close as possible, focus once more on your intention. As you come, send out this energy through the crown of your head and through your body, feeling the energies of Sol and Luna coursing through you. Then, if you feel up for it, ingest (or anoint yourself with) your own sexual fluids, and feel this elixir moving through your body, lighting you up from the inside out, knowing that the Sun and the Moon are present within you.

Stay in the afterglow for as long as you'd like and need.

Step 7: Declaration of alchemical union, dismissal of Sol and Luna

Once you feel ready, stand before your altar once again. You may perform a declaration of the working being finished before dismissing Sol and/or Luna by saying something like the following:

I/We now declare that the Divine Union of Sol and Luna through the erotic alchemical Path of Temperance is complete, the working finished, and sent forth to the highest.

If you invoked Sol, you may add:

Oh, Sol, embodied through Beauty, luminary of the heart and center of all, seat of wisdom and consciousness, I thank you for imbuing me with your Divine radiance for this working. The ritual is closed, and the working is complete. You are free to leave at peace. Blessed be.

Feel the Sun's golden light moving up through your body and back into the cosmos.

If you invoked Luna, you may add:

Oh, Luna, embodied through the Foundation, luminary of intuitive wisdom and understanding, seat of the mysteries and subconscious, I thank you for imbuing me with your Divine presence for this working. The ritual is closed, and the working is complete. You are free to leave at peace. Blessed be.

After you say this, feel the Moon's silver light moving up through your body and back into the cosmos.

Now thank the Path of Temperance/Samekh for the guidance and support. You may say something like the following as you stand before the Temperance card:

Oh, Temperance, the erotic alchemist, thank you for blessing us with this working of Divine Union of Sol and Luna. The ritual is done, and the working is complete. All energies are free to leave. Blessed be.

Step 8: Close and ground

Feel the profundity of the working moving through you. Breathe, and then perform your closing grounding and centering exercises. Feel all celestial energies move back into the cosmos above and all terrestrial energies into the earth below. Press your forehead into the earth, and flow any lingering energies back into Gaia. Thank yourself and your partner, and record the ritual and any feelings it brought up in your grimoire. Be sure to drink water, eat something, and ground into your body.

Allow the candles to burn all the way down, leaving them in the sink if necessary. If you need to extinguish the flame, use a candle snuffer or a fan rather than blowing them out. Relight them the next time you want to connect to your intention. Dispose of any excess wax in a garbage can at an intersection. And so it is.

CHAPTER 6

The Path of Divine Union

If Eros is the connective tissue of the universe, then love brings it an iridescent essence. If Eros is the form, then love is the force. This isn't to say that love has to be present for sex to be sacred. If there's one intention I hold very highly, it's *not* to repackage the patriarchal beliefs of the Church in a new age glamour. Sex can be sacred in whatever way makes sense to you, and love can be an imbibing force without needing to be *in love*. Love is a state of being in complete surrender with the Divine Will, and when this is honored alongside an exploration of sex, one is walking the Path of Divine Union.

The Path of Divine Union is for those who engage in sacred sex as a part of a committed relationship, as a portal to divine connectedness that can only be shared when sex becomes a ritual sacrament. It doesn't matter whether you're married, dating, in a long-term relationship, monogamous, or polyamorous; it is only the strength and honesty of your devotion that is important. Like the Path of

Alchemy, the Path of Divine Union requires complete trust and surrender in both seeing and being seen. Yet this path also can be walked by those who are not in an earthly relationship but wish to dedicate themselves to a deity, the cosmos, or their higher sexual self.

The through line is love. Love of the other, of the self, or of the Divine. Love is the connective tissue. It is the catalyst for ecstasy and a direct link to something greater. The guiding archetypal force for this path is the Lovers, the sixth key of the tarot. The Path of Divine Union aims to rectify the duality inherent in the self, the polarity of shadow and light, of perceived good and evil, of yin and yang, of solar and lunar, of expansion and contraction. The Path of Divine Union can even rectify the imbalance of certain aspects of the self, like if you feel your head and your heart are uneasy grounds and one is always leading the way. Thomas Moore says that, "Sex with soul is always a communion with another level of existence," and when woven with intention, we have the potential for true magick. This is an especially potent journey if you are married or in a long-term committed relationship that you wish to tend to like a vibrant garden.

The Path of Divine Union is all about shedding the illusion of separation and merging together as one. When it's in the container of a conscious relationship, empathy, awareness, and gnosis bubble to the surface of the cosmic interweaving of souls and bodies. This is a path that caters to those who are in a sacred relationship, who have made the commitment to love together, grow together, and totally and completely examine their shit together. This means releasing the tendency many of us have to pacify the difficult things that come up when two people bring their hearts and worlds together, and instead see everything as an opportunity to heal and intensify the dynamic. This is also alchemical work! Sex is the ritual that rectifies these moments of intensity, vulnerability, and pain.

You also may explore this path as a means of attaining the knowledge and conversation with the Holy Guardian Angel (HGA). The HGA is the higher self that is both separate from the self and a part of it, the cosmic lover that supports the magician in their accomplishment of the Great Work. Allow your life, your circumstances, your beliefs, and your desires to guide you in crafting the path that feels right *for you*.

THE SACRED TENETS OF CONSCIOUS RELATIONSHIP

The cookie-cutter idea of what a sacred union should look like (monogamous, heterosexual, vanilla) isn't going to be the right format for everyone. I have come to the realization that I am more interested in a relationship with a container of connection and communication built around it, instead of trying to squeeze into a mold or label that doesn't fit.

One couple I consider a shining example of this tenant are Haven and Sebastian, whom I met at a sex party they cohosted. Haven and Sebastian have been married for eight years and each have a child from a previous marriage. Their relationship is rooted in adventure, in saying yes, and in expanding their consciousness through psychedelics. Over the years I have known them, they have become muses, friends, lovers, and models of nurturing a Divine Union while juggling the responsibilities of full-time jobs, families, and life.

I asked Haven and Sebastian what it means for them to be in a conscious relationship—the foundation for any sort of Divine Union. Haven told me, "honesty and transparency, vulnerability, and realness." Sebastian said that a conscious relationship is "one where I'm constantly vigilant to never be taking anything for granted or throwing it into cruise control. You're conscious of the way you show up, the words you say, the way you act, the way you take accountability for your own actions, the way you hold your partner accountable for their actions—they're all done with intentionality."

One way to conceptualize this is by expanding the definition of what a "successful" relationship is. For Haven and Sebastian, everything is offered up, which means conversation around each other's comfort and needs is constant and ongoing. "By being in a conscious relationship where we are each our whole authentic selves, then we can courageously and fearlessly show up like that for our partner," Sebastian explains. "It unlocks a whole spectrum of excitement and adventure and intrigue in sex because nothing is out of bounds, no exploration is not on the table." For them, this meant expanding the notion that success included monogamy.

This trust, devotion, and freedom guided them toward a deeper sense of sovereignty and self-awareness. "Since he and I have been together, and we have committed ourselves, I have felt personally freer and more independent than I ever have in my whole adult life," Haven explains. "I'm willing to jump in and try it out because I know somebody who has my back. I know I have somebody who would never shame me, who would only encourage me to explore, not only as an individual but as a couple."

Whether you're monogamous, in an open relationship, polyamorous, or anyplace else on the relationship spectrum, your relationship should be built for you and your beloved with a foundation that honors you both.

EXAMPLES OF DIVINE UNION

Another way of honoring the Path of Divine Union is by connecting to the mythos and stories that represent this journey, both in fiction and in real life. What this means is noticing and admiring couples and relationships, whether magickal or mundane, that inspire a sort of soul-longing within you. In my own life, that includes both the sacred partnership of the Gods I worship and the Divine Unions of human beings like occultists Jack Parsons and Marjorie Cameron, musicians Poison Ivy and Lux Interior of the Cramps, and designers Vivienne Westwood and Andreas Kronthaler. I also have friends, like Haven and Sebastian, who inspire the sort of conscious relationship I want one day. Each of the relationships I admire, no matter how imperfect, teaches me about what I do and don't want in a sacred partnership.

Here are some examples of Divine Unions from different myths, cultures, and traditions. If you are already in a sacred part-nership, take the time to study and explore these examples—and your own—with your partner as a way of creating a personal mythos or blueprint for your relationship.

Shakti and Shiva: In Hindu tradition, Shakti and Shiva rep-resent creative consciousness manifested through the Divine Union. "The universe is a manifestation of play or polariza-tion between Shakti and Shiva" which is reflected in the life force or "prana" of the body.

Shekinah and God: The union of God and the feminine face of the Divine in the mystic Jewish tradition is exemplified through the Shekinah. The term originally referred to the "aspect of deity that can be apprehended by the senses," but in Talmudic tradition, Shekinah is seen as a reflection of feminine force, analogous to Shakti. The union of God and Shekinah is reflected in the mitzvah or sacred commandment of a married couple having sex on the Sabbath.

Nuit and Hadit: In the Thelemic worldview, the religion created by Aleister Crowley, Divine Union is represented by the deities Nuit and Hadit, two of its three central deities. Nuit is the limitlessness of the soul, expressed as the stars in the night sky, and her consort, Hadit, is embodied sexual force, the point to Nuit's circumference, representing the physical personification of Nuit's limitlessness.

Jesus and Mary Magdalene: Up until the time of Jesus, the Great Work of mysticism and self-evolution was only taken upon by the proverbial 1 percent, but his work and sacrifice generated a light or rainbow bridge for others to follow. Mary was Jesus's most beloved disciple and as passed down through the channeling of *The Magdalen Manuscript*, it's through practicing sex magick with Mary that Jesus was able to lay the foundation for egalitarian enlightenment. Mary was the feminine activating force, the Shakti energy, that allowed Jesus the ability to complete his purpose or True Will.

THE LOVERS AND DIVINE UNION

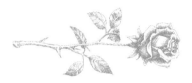

Even if you're unfamiliar with the Tarot, you'd likely recognize the Lovers, or the sixth key of the major arcana. It shows a man and a woman in the Garden of Eden, with an angel blessing them from above. The human figures are naked, with the man gazing at the woman and the woman gazing at the angel.

The Lovers represent the self-conscious and subconscious coming together in Divine Union to birth the super consciousness, which is represented by Raphael, the angel of the sphere of Tiferet/Beauty on the Tree of Life. When two disparate aspects of self come together, new perspectives and dimensions are possible. The Path of Divine Union leads to the integration of these mental states, through using the beloved as a mirror to view new aspects of the self.

So what does this have to do with sex? The Lovers speak of levels of consciousness that are intimately tied to the sexual self, and new realms are revealed through the shedding of clothes and coming together of bodies. One of my favorite quotes about the Lovers comes from Rachel Pollack, in her classic book on tarot, *Seventy-Eight Degrees of Wisdom*: "Through love, we not only achieve a unity with someone else, but we are given a glimpse of the greater meanings and deeper significance of life. In love we give up part of the ego control which isolates us not only from other people but from life itself. Therefore the angel appears above the man's and woman's heads, a vision unobtainable to each person individually, but glimpsed by both of them together." When the inner Sun and Moon merge in this way, you're able to ascend to a greater height. When you do this through the flesh, the individual bodies literally become unified.

The secret here is that even if you're walking the Path of Divine Union with another, what this mirrors is your inner Divine Union. This path requires that your lover mirrors your deepest truth and, thus, reflects the rectification of duality taking place within you. It's almost a union in three parts: your inner union, your lover's inner union, and the union of you both. The union of each individual acts as the two ends of a bridge, and the intention of sexual gnosis and evolution marries you.

JOURNAL QUESTIONS

The Path of Divine Union is felt as a soul yearning for embodied love through the flesh of the beloved. Relationships of any kind take work and introspection. And sometimes it's when you're so caught up in the intense sensations of Divine Union that taking pen to paper can help you come back to reality. At the very least, having a record will be a timestamp of the relationship, a way to remember being caught up in Divine Love, and a wonderful memory to have in years to come.

Set up your space as laid out in Chapter 1, decide if you want to answer these alongside your beloved, and then get to it!

- What do you think of when you hear "Divine Union"? What does this bring up? How has this changed or evolved since reading this chapter?
- What does conscious and sacred relationship mean to you?
- What does it mean for you to walk the Path of Divine Union alongside your beloved? The Divine? Yourself?
- What sexual experiences have helped you feel Divine Union?
- How does honoring all aspects of your sexuality and erotic essence allow you to show up more fully, whether for yourself, the Divine, or the beloved?
- How do your desires bring you closer to Divine Union?
- How do the Path of Alchemy and the Path of Divine Union complement each other?
- How does devotion help guide you in the mysteries of sex? How does this show up for you in a relationship or relationships?
- How does seeing the Divine in your beloved remind you of the Divine in yourself?
- What are some examples of couples in your life and in pop culture who walk the Path of Divine Union? What do they speak of to you? How do they help guide you?
- Are there any myths of Gods and Goddesses who inspire you to walk this path?

A TAROT SPREAD FOR RADIATING DIVINE LOVE INTO THE WORLD

You walk the path of sacred sex to know yourself more fully, to find meaning in the flesh and in the sensual, and to bring this to your lovers and the universe. This tarot spread will help you understand how to take the Path of Divine Union with you out into the world—and how to deal with these human issues that come up as you do this work.

Center yourself in any way you see fit. Perform the grounding and shielding exercises in the beginning of this book, or any other rituals that bring you a sense of centeredness and love, and set up yourself and your space. Ask your cards a specific question around how to radiate love, or simply ask what you need to know as you move forward on this path. Shuffle the cards, draw, and interpret, recording your results in your grimoire alongside any observations, downloads, and feelings. And so it is.

> *Card 1:* How can I embody Divine Union?
> *Card 2:* How can I share this with others or my beloved?
> *Card 3:* How can I radiate Divine Love outward in all I do?
> *Card 4:* How can I continue to choose love even when
>   feelings like jealousy or insecurity come up?
> *Card 5:* What's my message from the Universe for this path?

AFFIRMATIONS

No matter what path you walk, shit eventually will hit the fan. And so it's true with the Path of Divine Union, *especially if you're walking this path alongside someone you're in a conscious relationship with.* Taking the time to refocus and reframe at your own pace and time is every-thing, and affirmations can help you remember *why* you com-mitted to this work to begin with. Whether you're moving closer to your higher sexual self or making a commitment to your beloved, affirmations can support you when it feels difficult and draining. Allow them to remind you of the beauty of devotion, and how Divine Love is there for you when life feels overwhelming. Use the steps in Chapter 1 to make the most of your affirmations.

- I am Divine Love.
- I walk the Path of Divine Union.
- I honor the sacred marriage within myself.
- I am my own beloved.
- I walk the path of sacred and conscious relationship.
- I honor the unity of all my Divine dualities.
- My sexuality guides me deeper into Divine Union.
- My erotic essence guides me deeper into Divine Love.
- The more I honor my fullest expression, the more I honor my beloved.
- I honor my beloved through our sacred partnership.
- I honor the lunar and solar within me.
- I rectify all dualities through the alchemical furnace of love.
- Divine Love guides me and holds me.
- The Divine Erotic inspires and guides me.
- I am fully present in the sensual experiences of life.
- Feelings of pain and fear lead me back to love.

A CONSECRATION RITUAL OF DIVINE UNION

To undergo initiation into Divine Union is a big step. It is a sacred commitment, not an unbreakable bond, but a soul-centered one that risks pain and vulnerability in the name of love. This isn't something to rush into, and my suggestion is that this be undertaken only by couples who are committed to one another and to engaging in a sacred relationship. This ritual also can be undertaken by someone who is committing to their own Divine Union within the self, or as a devotional commitment to a deity or the cosmos/universe.

This ritual works with cleansing and consecration, with sex magick, and with sexual fluids, and it honors the act of sacred sex as an entry point into Divine Union. It is best performed during a new or waning Moon as a way to begin a new journey. You may perform it on a Friday, the day of Venus, for an extra dose of Divine Love.

What you need: Water (tap water, Moon water, rose water, Florida water, etc.), anointing oil (high-grade olive oil, frankincense oil, sandalwood oil, rose oil, ylang ylang oil, or jasmine oil), sacred herbs to burn (lavender, mugwort, cedar, ethically sourced palo santo), a lighter and container for the herbs, your Sacred Sex Grimoire, and any sex toys or lube. *If you are performing this ritual solo, you will need a mirror.*

Before you begin this ritual, read it over and meditate on what this rite of passage means to you. Think about your partner, or yourself, and how making this commitment will change your relationship and elevate it to the spiritual realm. This means that even when you're engaging in nonmagickal sex (aka sex for fun and not as part of a ritual or working), *it will still be sacred because the whole relationship becomes sacred after passing through this portal.* You may work with the journal questions and tarot spread earlier in this chapter as well. If you are doing this ritual with a partner, talk about what it means for both of you and how it will change your relationship.

If you want to erect an altar specific to this ritual, place flowers like roses, the Lovers tarot card, photos, jewelry, letters, icons, and anything else that represents your Divine Union on it. If you are engaging with this ritual with a partner or partners, you may each add something that represents you.

You will need to know what direction is east before you begin.

Step 1: Get ready
If you are doing this partnered, give each other space until the ritual begins. Take a shower or bath, adorn yourself in your favorite ritual wear and jewels, and put on perfume if you like. Set up the space per usual.

Step 2: Enter the temple and ground and shield
As you enter the temple, see it as opening the door to your heart, to your beloved or self or the Divine. Light any candles or incense that correlate to your intention. Gaze at your beloved and the altar. Then find a comfortable position across from your beloved; close your eyes; and take a moment to ground, shield, and center (page 38).

Now meditate on your heart center. Feel the Divine light from below and above meeting here, and draw it into your heart. Notice how spacious or closed off it feels; the point is not to judge, not to theorize, not to change, *but just to notice the state of your heart and give it love and compassion.*

When you feel ready, you will cleanse and consecrate, using water and fire. If you are doing this ritual with a partner or partners, assign someone to the water and someone to the fire. Or you may wish to do both together.

Grab your water and, starting in the east, sprinkle it before you as you say:

Through the waters of the most sacred heart

Then move a quarter turn to the right so you're facing the south, and sprinkle water before you as you say:

Through the portal of erotic intuition

Once again, move a quarter turn to the right so you're facing the west, and sprinkle water before you as you say:

I cleanse this temple

Finally, move a quarter turn to the right so you're facing the north, and sprinkle water before you as you say:

In the name of Divine Love

When you're done, anoint your partner(s) or yourself with the water and have your partner(s) anoint you, too. Start at the crown of the head, then the third eye, the higher heart, the solar plexus, and the sacral center under the belly button. Feel this anointing remove any worry, fears, baggage, or any energy that doesn't vibrate in 100 percent Divine light.

Now you will be following the same pattern with fire.

Light your herbs and then blow them out so there's just the smolder of smoke.

Begin facing the east, and fan the smoke before you as you say:

Through the fires of fiercest devotion

Then move a quarter turn so you're facing the south, and fan the smoke before you as you say:

Through the portal of erotic commitment

Once again, move a quarter turn so you're facing the west, and fan the smoke before you as you say:

I consecrate this temple

Then move a quarter turn so you're facing the north, and fan the smoke before you as you say:

In the name of Divine Union

Now that you've consecrated the space, cleanse your partner(s) or yourself with the sacred smoke, beginning at the top of the head and moving through each part of the body, including the arms and legs, the torso, the palms, the bottoms of the feet, and between the legs. Feel it burning away anything stopping you from aligning with the Divine and with your union.

If you are honoring this Divine Union
by dedicating yourself to a deity, now is the time
to invoke them and invite them into your ritual.

Step 3: Eye-gaze

It's time to form the divine connection you are consecrating today through eye-gazing or mirror-gazing. If there is an odd number of participants, set a timer and switch after a while so everyone eye-gazes with everyone else. If you are participating in this ritual solo, you will be eye gazing into a mirror.

Find a comfortable position across from your partner. Set a timer for three to five minutes. Place their right hand over your heart and your left hand over your partner's right hand, and have them do the same. Take a few deep breaths into your heart center as you match inhales and exhales with each participant. Then, gaze into your partner's left eye, or your own in the mirror, as you continue to breathe. Allow this to be silly and awkward if it is, *but don't talk.* The silence is the void in which the cosmic egg is hatching. If this turns into a visionary experience, breathe into it, but stay in the body as much as you can.

If you are doing this with an odd number of people, repeat as many times as needed so everyone eye-gazes with everyone else.

Step 4: Anoint and affirm

Now you will be anointing one another, or yourself, with oil as you declare your intention. With your oil by your side, put a tiny amount on your fingertips and anoint it on the forehead of your beloved as you gaze into their eyes, or on your own forehead as you gaze in the mirror, if you're doing this alone. The partner being anointed, or you if you're doing this alone, should say:

I open myself up on all planes in all ways to the dance of Divine Union with [the name of your partner(s), yourself, your deity, etc.].

Anoint the throat next and say:

May my soul, my words, my heart, and my actions reflect this sacred commitment to Divine Union

Anoint the higher heart next and say:

I commit to this initiation into Divine Union on all planes in all ways. I open myself up to you, in all planes in all ways. I perform this ritual of the sacred marriage of body and soul, in all planes in all ways. For the highest good of all involved, in alignment with my True Will. And so it is.

If you are doing this with a partner or partners, repeat this process, having the partner who was just anointed do this on the other partner. After everyone has been anointed, you will all say together:

I am divided for love's sake, for the chance of union.

Step 5: Make love, and raise the energy

Begin exploring the physicality of the flesh. Work with touch, kissing, and massage to raise the erotic energy in the room. Whisper words of gratitude and love to yourself or to the other. Allow this sacred foreplay to remind you of why you're doing this ritual.

You may begin in the position known as "yab yum," where both partners face one another, with one partner on the lap of the other, and both have their legs loosely wrapped around the other. This way, your spines will stay straight, which helps with the flow of energy, and you're able to make eye contact and kiss while your hearts and flesh press into one another. You can also begin in any sexual position in which you and your partner face each other.

Before you have sex, take a moment to sit in this energy. The threshold you're about to pass through is shimmering before you. Take a moment to recognize how *huge* this commitment is. As you begin having sex, match your movements to your breath, allowing it to guide your pace. Feel yourself moving into Divine Union with each breath, with each thrust, with each touch.

As you feel yourself and/or your partner orgasm, make eye contact and send the energy into each other. Repeat this visualization with eye contact as necessary for each person involved. If you are fluid bound, any partners with a penis may ejaculate; the semen will be used in the following step. If you are doing this by yourself, gaze into the mirror or just feel the energy penetrating your auric body and circulating through you.

No matter if you're performing this ritual solo or partnered,
know that this orgasm or this raising of energy
is creating a divine link between you and the other.
This is an energetic manifestation of your sacred vow
to partnership, and it is holy as fuck.

After, take a moment to lie with your beloved or yourself, feeling the energy moving through you, visualizing how you want to embody this new stage of your relationship. Be here as long as you need.

Step 6: Consecrate the initiation

Affirm the initiation by consecrating your beloved(s) or yourself with your sexual fluids. These represent your transformed essence. Taking sexual fluids from the vagina or penis, anoint yourself or your beloved on the forehead, throat, and heart and then lick your fingers and have your partner do the same. The partner being anointed may say:

> *I now affirm this initiation into sacred union. I come out transformed, and whole unto myself, through the power of sacred sexuality and Divine Love. The two have become one. The working is complete, but the Divine Union is everlasting. And so it is.*

Repeat with each partner, and speak whatever words flow from your heart.

Step 7: Close the working

Sit in meditation for a moment and reconnect to your heart. Notice what feels different—is it softer, more expansive, more full? Surrender to whatever feelings come up, and notice how the Divine Union has already allowed you the opportunity to grow and evolve. Close and ground, and thank and dismiss any deities that were called in. Press your forehead into the ground, and send any excess energy back into the earth.

Take notes in your grimoire, and spend time with yourself, your partner, or your deity in front of your altar, in prayer or meditation, or in conversation. Know that this is just the beginning, and that the real work is what comes after. May this path open new worlds of love and connection.

CHAPTER 7

The Path of the Mystic

S ex as an art of devotion, as a means of embodying and entwining with the Divine Feminine. Sacred sexuality as a sacrament to the highest, as a connection to the ancient egregore of the Temple Priestess, the sacred slut, the holy whore. This is the Path of the Mystic; this is the Path of the Hetaera; this is the Path of the Erotic Votary.

The Goddess of Love in her many guises is honored through the flesh. In the ancient past, the Priestesses of the Goddess of Love honored her through their own sexual energy, expression, and the act of sex itself. Not only was the Priestess acting as and embodying the Goddess, she was offering up her own sexual energy as well, while also transmitting this frequency to whomever she was in ceremony with. These erotic votaries—or "sacred prostitutes" as many call them—may or may not have actually existed. But as magickal practitioners and sex witches, we know the *current*, the magickal force, is most definitely real. The way of the sacred slut and holy whore is open before you.

The Path of the Mystic and Erotic Votary is defined by engaging with sex and sexual energy as a doorway to the Divine Feminine, and more specifically to this erotic and life-giving force in her guise as Goddess of Love. Sex and sex magick become a means of connecting with the Divine in and through the self. When this is carried out with authenticity and devotion, sex itself becomes communion with the Goddess.

Of all of the paths in this book, the is the one I relate to most. Sex, sexuality, and the Divine Erotic are ways in which I honor, connect with, and embody the Goddess of Love and Lust. Masturbation becomes a ritual of offering energy. Dating becomes an invitation to embrace the Babalonian and Venusian within me. Sexuality turns into the slithering and vibrating force that reminds me of my commitment to the Goddesses I serve. My sexuality is my own, yet it's also a force outside myself, guiding me through this life in service of the Goddess of Love.

THE EROTIC VOTARY
IN THE ANCIENT PAST

The earliest known poet in recorded history, Enheduanna (who was a High Priestess of the Goddess of Sex and War, Inanna) lived in ancient Sumer approximately 4,200 years ago. Inanna's myth is written in erotic terms, and her priestess expresses longing and lust for her Goddess. This is where we get the term *Hierodule*, which means "sacred servant" and denotes religious officials whose rites include the sexual act. Inanna's successor, Ishtar, was called the Great Goddess Har, Mother of Harlots. Inanna, Ishtar, Anath, Astarte, Isis,

Cybele, Venus, and Aphrodite were likewise said to have Temple Priestesses who engaged in sexual ritual as part of their responsibilities to the Goddess of Love and her temple: "Wherever the goddess of fertility, love, and passion was worshipped, the sacred prostitute was an integral member of the community," notes the book *The Sacred Prostitute: Eternal Aspect of the Feminine.*

The erotic votaries may be called sacred sluts, holy whores, or Temple Priestesses. If you are engaging with your sexuality in a similar manner and using it as an offering and guiding connection to the Goddess, you may even adopt one or more of these titles. (This may feel especially potent if you are a sex worker.) The more you embrace the name of sacred slut or holy whore, the less negative power it has over you. Sex and spirit have been intertwined since the beginning of time, and it's time to reclaim this divine symbiosis.

The erotic votary weaves a spell of desire and lust. Eroticism becomes the connective tissue, the conduit, the antenna to which the gross and subtle body are attuned. Sexuality is the socket and the electricity. Sex becomes the current that connects to the Divine. This current is embodied as Kundalini and in the tantrikas of the Left Hand Path of tantra. The taboo against sex is part of the reason there is so much power in breaking this boundary. *There can be no transgression without taboo.*

THE EROTIC VOTARY TODAY

You don't have to be devoted to a specific face of the Goddess or even to the Goddess at all to walk the Path of the Mystic. You can work with sex as a sacrament to source or to God because *it's the immanence* in this relationship that defines your devotion. On the Path of the Mystic, the body is the temple, and the heart is the altar. The Divine is both within and without, in everyone and everything. Sex becomes more than an act; it becomes a golden halo that surrounds your life. This is the Divine Erotic. Honoring the pursuit of the ecstatic and pleasure-filled as a means of affirming the unknowable enchants life with a glimmering aura. Any moment or act can become orgasmic— the feeling of the silk on bare skin, the sound of the birds, the whispering of a lover in your ear . . . everything becomes a portal into the realm of the cosmos. Everything has the potential to be a ritual of devotion. Sex becomes part of your spiritual practice, whether it's solo or partnered.

This path invites you to deepen your connection to sexual energy through meditation and ritual so you can immerse yourself erotically with more control and reverence. Professional dominatrix, clinical hypnotherapist, sex witch, and Goddess devotee Sydney Jones says, "The Goddess is in you, it's everywhere. I just want people to realize that these things are really powerful, they're really powerful catalysts, they're powerful catalysts for change, they're powerful catalysts for self-growth and connection to what is really divine, even if society is trying to tell you it's not."

Embracing the sacred slut and holy whore, the Path of the Mystic and Erotic Votary includes accepting all sorts of sexualities. It means sex positivity—supporting an individual's choice of sexual expression and embodiment, no matter how different it is from your own. It is all about radical erotic self-awareness and sex as a devotional offering to the Divine, the other, and the self.

THE MYSTIC AND
THE CYCLES OF THE MOON

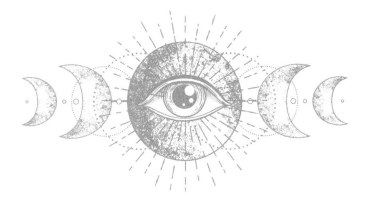

This path is sensual and cyclical. It is fluid and ever-evolving, attuned to the currents of sexual energy in the body and how it flows through you. One method to sync your energy is by working with the lunar cycles. The Moon is an ancient source of power that has been around for more than 4.5 billion years. Simply contemplating the fact that every single person who has ever existed has gazed up at the same moon is enough to inspire a state of awe.

In astrology, the Moon represents the depths of the psyche, the unconscious, and the fertile and generative forces of creation as expressed by the Divine Feminine. In the natal chart, or the astrological snapshot of where all the planets were at your exact time of birth, the Moon represents your inner world, the way you like to be nurtured and cared for, your relationship with your mother, and your hidden but true self. As astrologer extraordinaire Amelia Quint shares, "The sun is your identity, and the moon is emotions, and I think that whether we like it or not with sexuality, feelings and emotions and the body can come into play, so I think the Moon can be a piece of it."

Each month, the Moon goes through a death and rebirth, mimicking the renewal of the uterine lining of those who menstruate. At the beginning of its twenty-eight-day cycle, the Moon is inky black with no light from the Sun reflected on its surface. As it waxes, its light grows and grows until the peak of its potency and power at the full Moon, the energetic climax (or orgasm) of the month. Then the Moon wanes, or loses light, until the cycle begins again.

Sympathetic magick, or magick that imitates its desired outcome, is a way to honor this by working to manifest something as the light of the Moon grows, from new to full Moon, and working to release something as it shrinks from full to new. Although I will begin by sharing how to work with Luna starting in her new Moon phase, you can jump into this practice at any phase.

THE NEW MOON: PLANTING SEEDS OF EROTIC INTENTION

The new Moon is when you get the chance to cocreate with the cosmos. Because there is no light from the Sun reflected on the Moon, this is a moment to tread the psychic and dark waters of the self.

The new Moon is like key zero in the tarot, the Fool. It's an energy of new beginnings that requires trust and surrender, and this is when you can align with your intention and vision to carry it forward through the month. Sexually, the new Moon is the time to plant seeds of erotic intent. This would be like the negotiation stage of a BDSM scene, or sexting ahead of a date to tease and decide what sort of sex is going to take place. This is when you ask yourself what your fantasies are, what sort of experiences you'd like, how you want to make love, how you can offer this to the Goddess, and what you want to get out of your moment. For the erotic votary, this is when you decide what sort of ritual setting you'd want to engage in, what sort of offerings you want to include, and what the intention for this will be.

This is most likely when you'll begin your devotional, or a period of time in which an ongoing ritual is held in service to a desire. (You will be led in creating a sacred sex devotional later in this chapter.) The new Moon reflects the opening of this devotional, the intention setting and initiatory ritual. Think of the first kiss, the first touch, the first flirt. It's when your eyes lock with your lover and you feel electricity coursing between you. In your solo sexual practice, the new Moon is when you breathe into your own sexual energy.

THE WAXING MOON: THE TIME OF ENERGETIC FOREPLAY

The waxing Moon is when your intentions and desires grow. You begin to tend to your life to feed into your intention, both in your magickal practice and mundane existence. On the Path of the Erotic Mystic, the waxing Moon is like energetic foreplay: the making out and heavy petting and 69ing. In a ritual setting, it is when you raise energy. You can do this through breath work, masturbation, and sex. This is also when you gather energy for your devotional and strengthen your connection to Goddess through feeding her energy, dedication, and time.

THE FULL MOON:
THE PEAK OF ECSTASY

The full Moon is Luna's orgasm, when all the building of light and energy reaches its climax. This is the time of your fullest connection to your erotic power. In sex, this is when you embody your fullest divinity and become one with the Goddess or the beloved. In a devotional context, this is when you can use orgasms to feed your intention. The full Moon is when you take all the energy you've raised and send this to the cosmos to manifest your intention. This is already two weeks after the new Moon, so this may also mark the completion of this long-form ritual, unless you continue it to the next new Moon (or for as long as you want).

The full Moon is when you get to connect to yourself as an erotic votary, as a sacred mystic of sex. This is the time of sex magick, of working with the power of orgasm to catalyze change on the physical plane or as a means of channeling, embracing, and connecting with your sexual power. During this phase, you can work with sexual fluids like semen, vaginal secretion, or menstrual blood and saliva to consecrate talismans, anoint magickal tools and weapons or statues or icons of deities, and anoint and consecrate yourself and lovers. The full Moon is when you come back to yourself as a sexual Priest/ess, committed to owning every aspect of who you are, without shame, judgment, or diminishment of your erotic strength.

THE WANING MOON:
THE TIME OF AFTERGLOW AND INTEGRATION

After the peak of the full Moon, as the Moon wanes or loses light, you bask in the energetic afterglow. This is a period of integration, when you allow yourself to release and rest. In sex, this is the post-coital stage, when you bond with yourself and your lover through touch, taste, and sound. In a devotion, this means giving offerings and gratitude after you finished your working on the full Moon, or it would be a period of sustained dedication through sex magick and worship.

THE DARK MOON:
THE TIME OF REFLECTION AND THE DARK GODDESS

The Dark Moon is the last aspect of the lunar cycle, and some witches don't distinguish it from the waning or new Moon. The Dark Moon is the days before the new Moon, when there is no light on the Moon. This is a time of parting ways with your lover, cleaning up your mess, or coming back to a normal state of consciousness as the afterglow wears off. In ritual, this would be the days after the working is done, when you take the time to notice its effects. Your devotional may not be complete if you're working from new Moon to new Moon, but this is still a time of final offerings and finishing the cycle.

The Dark Moon is also a portal to the arcane mysteries of sex and death as represented by the Dark Goddess. This is the Goddess of the shadow and subversive, who guides you into the unexplored crevices of the self. She asks that you honor your sexuality openly and honestly. Notice what has shifted exoterically in the outer world and esoterically in the internal realms. This is a time to honor whatever pain, fear, or sadness has shifted or that has come up since you've made more space for yourself through this devotional. Find peace with the shadow and cultivate a relationship with it, even if it's painful.

This is also when you record the results of your working in your grimoire, when you commune with your deity or Goddess or partner and ask, "Was this as good for you as it was for me?" You may be feeling tender, sensitive, and in an altered state of consciousness. The Dark Moon induces space for that, so bask in the vortex of transformation.

THE PATH OF THE MYSTIC, NEOTANTRA, AND KUNDALINI

The Path of the Mystic is an amalgamation of frameworks of sexual devotion. The current runs through Temple Priestess and erotic votaries of the ancient past, as well as through the tradition of tantra in the East and sexual magick in the West. When these currents meet, they result in "neotantra," which is the sort of tantra those of you in the Western world are most familiar with. As you already learned, the tantrikas, or initiates of a tantric lineage, perform complex rituals to "recognize the essential essence of Shakti or Divine Feminine energy" flowing through all things. It's when this life force has been activated that Shiva, or the Divine Masculine consciousness, can be awakened. Authentic tantra requires a disciplic relationship with a guru and a high-level understanding of Sanskrit because many rituals focus on visualizing and enshrining the physical and etheric bodies with Sanskrit letters, and as in Hebrew, these letters act as containers for specific energies. Beyond this, tantric rituals are long and complex.

Neotantra takes the sexual aspect of LHP tantra alongside sexual magick, as brought forth by Randolph, Crowley, and others, and the wisdom of the Kama Sutra to deliver something new. Long story short, tantra + sex magick = neotantra. Tantra without being initiated into a lineage by a guru, with a focus on sexual energy = neotantra. Sex magick seeks power, tantra seeks spiritual consciousness, and the erotic votary and sexual mystic works with sexual power as a means of attaining that illumination. The erotic mystic awakens this dormant aspect of the self through sex and the body.

The medium used to achieve illumination in this way is called Kundalini yoga. Kundalini is the Shakti energy of the exalted creative and Divine Feminine that resides at the base of the spine. This energy travels up two channels through the spine and central nervous system: the ida, or lunar/negative/left channel, is connected to the parasympathetic nervous system; and the pingala, or solar/active/right channel, is connected to the sympathetic nervous system. These channels, or nadis, spiral upward to the crown of the head, ending at the pineal gland, and act as conduits of Kundalini that feed the whole nervous system and subtle body. Kundalini yoga utilizes breath, sacred sounds like mantras and kirtan (chanting), hand gestures (mudras), energy locks (bandhas), and yoga postures (asanas) to accelerate the process of Kundalini rising up the spine, with the goal of attaining enlightenment *in this life*.

Part of the worship and adoration of tantra is that of the lingam, or penis, which represents Shiva, and the yoni, or vulva, which represents Shakti. The lingam is often seen as a cone or rod and the yoni as a hole. Together, they represent the balance of the Divine Feminine and Masculine forces.

Neotantra mixes these concepts with sacred sex and sex magick to establish a system that utilizes breath, movement, and sexual energy for a desired purpose, whether that's conscious sex, manifestation, or gnosis. Neotantra is a way of attaining ecstasy, both in the short term but also with the goal of the long term through the release of cycles of incarnation. Neotantra ritualizes breath work, bandhas or energy locks, eye-gazing, intention, ritual, and spell work to slow down the sexual act so it becomes numinous.

The Divine Feminine ties it all together. The Divine Feminine or Goddess is the latent erotic power that gives birth to everything—to the earth, to you, to your body, to the animals, to children, to creative projects. The Goddess creates, sustains, and destroys. The Goddess is both the abyss from all which life comes and the energy that allows it to manifest. *You* have this energy running through you—it's a frequency you can attune to. The Divine Feminine and Goddess energy aren't reliant on gender or sex. Your definition of Goddess will be personal, and fostering a relationship with her that fits into your life is potent stuff. But if this isn't an energy you vibe with, that's okay.

In the gnostic tradition, the feminine principle is manifested as Sophia, which means "wisdom." Wisdom is knowledge embodied, met with understanding, and used for illumination. In Qabalistic tradition, Sophia resides in the sphere or realm of Chokmah (Wisdom in Hebrew), while the Divine Feminine is seen in the sphere of Binah (Understanding). When these forces come together, they are reflected through Knowledge (Da'at), the secret sphere on the Tree of Life.

When you have an understanding of your sexuality, desires, kinks, body, and heart, and when you offer this knowledge to the Goddess, this becomes a way of experiencing her through the self. You become an emanation of the Goddess and closer to becoming the Divine yourself. As you dance and fuck your way through this path, you become a Priest/ess of Love. By creating devotionals and transforming yourself through sexual energy, you open to a new level of Eros, and to a new level of awareness. Through living erotically, and seeing your body as an energetic current, you become an antenna for the feminine, and a Priestess of Love to everyone you come into contact with.

THE HIGH PRIESTESS AS THE MUSE OF THE EROTIC VOTARY

The Path of the Divine Mystic works with devotion, neotantra, sex magick, and the Goddess as a spiritual framework. All your kinks, fetishes, and desires have space here, *and so does your heart*. The results are mind-blowing. One of the ways to begin your journey is to embrace the High Priestess, the second tarot key, correspondent to the luminary of the Moon. The High Priestess guards the mysteries passed from mouth to ear through initiation, gnosis, and soul exploration. She represents a middle way between the active and receptive, force and form, yin and yang, masculine and feminine. She exists outside of duality altogether.

In the classic Smith-Waite deck, the High Priestess sits between the black-and-white pillars of the Temple of Solomon, before the veil of knowledge. To pass through the mysteries, to move through the ceremony, requires a stillness found in the High Priestess. It's not enough to honor her; you must become her, finding a middle ground between force and form, sex and spirit. The High Priestess is the erotic gateway to the numinous, which must be experienced in the body and not just the mind.

The High Priestess is the inner light you tap into for illumination along the trip, like the Moon guiding you even in the dead of night.

But the light of the Priestess must be activated from within. The High Priestess is an embodiment of true wisdom, which is kept sub rosa (beneath the rose, only passed on to initiates) until those who can benefit from this knowledge prove themselves worthy.

The High Priestess is the initiatrix of the flesh, guarding the mysteries of sexuality until they can become enlightening forces in your own life. She does not speak, but expresses through the heart. She is not heard, but felt. The High Priestess asks you to pass through the veil into your own depths, to not logically assert your way to the Goddess of Love but to remember Her temple is ever existent at the portal of your heart. She is the holy whore of unconditional love who gives without expectation and reciprocity, who sees sex as a sacrament to all of life, and who invites you to adopt this view as well.

Now you are the Priestess. May you find strength and refuge in this magick.

TURNING ORGASMS INTO OFFERINGS

One of my favorite ways to tap into the matrix of the sacred slut is through devoting my sexual energy to the Goddess (or to a specific Goddess). Whether I'm engaging in some sacred solo sex or playing with a partner in a kink scene, transmuting my sexual energy into an offering is one way that I remain devoted to Goddess while also tapping into the erotic mysteries. Because this chapter is inspired by the erotic votaries of the ancient past, who worshipped the Goddesses of Love, working with a Goddess like Venus, Aphrodite, Babalon, Inanna, Astarte, Freya, Rati or Isis may resonate.

The practice of offering orgasms or sexual energy to Goddess is simple. When you masturbate or have sex, at orgasm or the peak of this climax, you send this charged energy through your body, directing it into the cosmos as an offering. You may visualize the deity or gaze at a statue, icon, or artistic depiction of the Goddess as you do. The fun of this is that you can make the process as elaborate as you want by working with correspondences like scent, color, adornment, sigils, and sacred symbols. If you're sending out energy to Venus, for example, you may wear rose perfume, burn rose incense, wear copper jewelry, or light green candles. If you're working with Isis, you may burn white candles and blue lotus incense, put on rose oil, and wear silver jewelry.

Spending time in meditation or prayer, communing with Goddess and developing a statement of intention around offering your orgasms, can enhance the ritual. When it comes time for the sexual element, slowing down and enjoying the sensations, breathing, making sounds and allowing vocal release, and basking is important. *This is devotion; this is offering.* As you worship Goddess in this way, you embody her. Take this practice as far as you want, anointing talismans, seals, sigils, or icons of the Goddess with sexual fluids or even inviting her to enter you before sex. As above, so below. As you offer your energy to the Divine Feminine, you offer it to yourself as well.

There are numerous energy centers in the body; most traditions work with five or seven. In Hindu and yogic traditions, these are known as chakras (which means "wheels" in Sanskrit). The chakras live along the spine. In the following table, find information about these energy centers, including their Sanskrit names, where on the spine they are located, and what they represent.

SEX MAGICK THROUGH THE CHAKRAS

CHAKRA	COLOR	LOCATION	CORRESPONDENCE
Muladhara	Red	Base of spine	Grounding, safety, security
Svadhisthana	Orange	A few inches below the belly button	Sexual energy, passion, life force
Manipura	Yellow	About four inches above the belly button	Confidence, willpower, strength
Anahata	Green	Heart/center of chest	Love, compassion, empathy
Vishuddha	Blue	Throat	Communication, clarity, your ability to express yourself
Ajna	Violet or indigo	Between the eyebrows	Spiritual visions, imagination, and seeing the truth of a situation
Sahasrara	Violet or white	Top of the head	Spiritual illumination, enlightenment, and cosmic consciousness

In the Western esoteric tradition, the energy centers run along the spine and correlate to the Middle Pillar on the Tree of Life. In Taoism, energy travels along the central channel as well as corresponding channels that move up the spine and throughout the body. In Chinese medicine, energy moves through what are called meridians, including along the spine. Different traditions give these energetic pathways different names, and many describe hundreds throughout the body.

The point is that this understanding of energetic flow isn't something that's just seen in one tradition, but in many. Deepening your sex magick practice requires you to be able to move energy up and through the body, and you can begin with breath work, visualization, and meditation.

Step 1: Masturbation meditation with the central channel

Start by masturbating and breathing energy up your spine to the crown of your head. You can try inhaling at the root chakra or pelvis and then exhaling as you send your awareness up to the crown of your head, or try leading your energy up the spine on an inhale and then returning your consciousness to the base of your spine with an exhale. Don't worry about the chakras or energy centers; just get used to the feeling of directing energy through the central channel and up your spine. As you reach climax, or as close as you can get, send this accumulated energy through the crown of your head into the cosmos to fulfill an intention, or circulate it back into your body to feel its life-sustaining energy.

Step 2: Masturbation meditation through the chakras

Once you've gotten the hang of directing energy up your spine, you'll begin to move through each chakra. To start, just hold your awareness at each center until you feel it's time to move to the next: first the root, then the sacral, the solar plexus, the heart, the throat, the third eye, and finally the crown. Try to time your orgasm so it happens as you reach the crown of your head. The more you do this, the more you'll notice how each energy center feels, transforms, and responds to the sexual vibration. At the root chakra it may feel heavy and grounding, while at the heart chakra, it may feel expansive and energizing.

It might also feel sticky or stuck, which indicates a block

around the themes this chakra reflects. In that case, try a separate meditation, sexual or otherwise, focusing on whichever center feels obstructed and feeding it white, healing energy and breath. For example, if you feel a blockage at the throat, this may indicate fear or resistance around speaking your truth and claiming your voice. Work with the planetary energy of Mercury, or a deity like Hermes or Thoth, as these are the planet and Gods of communication. Script affirmations that you repeat to yourself, especially during meditation, and burn orange candles, light lavender incense, and visualize the color orange infusing your throat chakra.

Step 3: Masturbation meditation through the chakras with visualization
Once you can feel the ways the different chakras transform your energy, visualize them as colors and symbols. You can use the classically associated colors for each chakra, and/or picture them as orbs, flowers, or wheels. As you breathe into each chakra, see it in its associated color, glowing, blooming, or spinning. I invite you to get familiar with the traditional associations and then devise your own.

JOURNAL QUESTIONS

One of the most beautiful aspects of committing to living a spiritual life, aligned with the cosmos and Divine Erotic, is the nonstop evolution. When you engage with your spiritual practice with curiosity and wonder, the learning and expansion never stops—and neither does the joy! Sexuality is an ever-running stream, and just when you think you know yourself completely, a new practice or partner leads you to a new experience, kink, feeling, or download. There is always more to learn, feel, explore, taste, and see. And so is this true on the Path of the Mystic and Erotic Votary.

Engaging with sacred sex through the lens of devotion has its specific quirks. Suddenly your sexuality is yours, but it also is something bigger. This can be overwhelming. The following journal questions are meant to help you find a solid foundation for your erotic devotion—and your heart. Use them as a jumping-off point for free writing, automatic writing, doodling, word association, or mind maps. Set up yourself and your space, and allow Goddess and your heart to guide you in this sacred unfolding.

- What does it mean to walk the Path of the Mystic?
- What does it mean to be an erotic votary or Temple Priestess? How do I swim in this current?
- What does it mean to me to honor my sexuality as something greater than myself?
- How do I relate my sexuality to the Divine Feminine?
- What does the Divine Feminine/Goddess mean to me?
- What are my experiences with Kundalini energy and erotic energy like? How do I feel this in my body?
- How can I explore neotantra as a path back into my body?
- How does seeing my sexual energy as something I can connect with, raise, dedicate, and offer deepen my relationship to this part of myself?
- What faces of the Divine do I connect with through this path?
- What sort of sensory experiences connect me to my sexuality and the numinous?
- What kind of rituals do I, or can I, create in my life that honor my sexuality and devotion?

- How can I see my body as an altar and temple to sacred sex?
- How can I work with my erotic self to embody and live as an incarnation of the Goddess?
- How can movement, breath, sound, and adornment help me further imbue Goddess energy into rituals of sacred sex?

A TAROT SPREAD
FOR AROUSING EROTIC DEVOTION

This tarot spread will help you walk the Path of the Erotic Votary with confidence and clarity, find guidance within yourself, and feel cosmically supported as you do so. No path is for everyone, but in a world that often rejects the Divine Feminine, it can be especially scary to surrender to this particular one. The cards offer perspective on the journey so you can remain as embodied, grounded, and protected as possible.

Turn this into as much of a ritual as you wish. As you feel ready, ask the cards what you need to know on this path, or something more specific. Then shuffle, pull, interpret, and record in your grimoire. And so it is.

Card 1: What does erotic devotion mean to me?
Card 2: How can I honor my sexuality as something that connects me to the Divine/Goddess/cosmos?
Card 3: How can I arouse this and carry it forward in my life?

Card 4: How can I remain protected and centered in myself as I do this?

Card 5: What do I need to know as I walk on the path of the erotic votary?

AFFIRMATIONS

To walk on the Path of the Mystic requires dedication both to yourself and to Goddess. One way you can remember this devotion is by claiming it out loud. Affirmations are like prayers, acting as anchors to the work whenever you need space and perspective. They are also a great tool to remind you of your *why*, and they can allow you to reorient with gratitude, sensuality, and joy.

Work with affirmations in ritual or as a part of a daily practice. Breathe into your heart and sexual center, feeling how energy flows between these two portals. Work with the steps laid out in Chapter 1 to make the most of this practice, and allow the Goddess to inspire you in writing your own affirmations.

- I am a Priestess of the Goddess.
- I am an erotic votary of love and magick.
- My sexuality and sexual expression are an offering to the cosmos.
- I offer my sexuality and orgasms to the Goddess.
- I am a conduit and channel for something larger than myself.
- I am an embodiment of love, lust, and magick.
- I walk the Path of the Sexual Mystic and Erotic Votary.

- I am devoted to my erotic self and to my sexual truth and magick.
- I share my sexual energy as a direct path to the Divine Feminine.
- I share my sexual energy and body with whomever I see fit.
- I am an expression of the Goddess, and I honor myself as such.
- I honor the sexual Priest/ess within myself through channeling the Divine Erotic.
- I come back to my fullest sensual and Divine expression on all planes, in all ways, always.

CREATING A
SACRED SEX DEVOTIONAL

One of my favorite magickal practices is a devotional. Devotionals are long-form rituals that take place over days, weeks, months, or even years. Although it is classically a period of worshipping a certain deity, a devotional can be anything you want to commit to in a magickal context, whether that's to drawing in love and sex, harnessing your subversive sexuality, or to the unknown. Forging this kind of vessel through a set period of time, and planning specific daily rituals and workings within it, is wildly powerful and profound and can usher in huge life changes and new states of being.

This is because during a devotional, even the mundane is transformed into magick. Everything you do, including day-to-day life outside the daily practices, becomes part of the work. A level of attention and awareness permeates the period in a really special way,

THE PATH OF THE MYSTIC

amplifying your intention much more than a single ritual or spell would.

For the erotic mystic, sex and sex magick become a focal point. You get to decide your intention, whether it is an offering or a means of self-exploration. Begin a sacred sex devotional that feels right for you. You may work with the tarot spread or journal questions earlier in this chapter to figure out the theme and intention of this devotional as well.

Step 1: Decide on your intention
Like any magickal working, the first step is always deciding the what or why. Before you can set up your space or do prep work, you need to know what you're prepping for. Here are some examples to consider:

MY INTENTION IS TO . . .

- Release shame and guilt around my sexual expression.
- Connect with the Goddess or a specific Goddess of Love or Lust and offer her my sexual energy.
- Connect with the erotic votary and Temple Priestess so I can embody this energy.
- Understand my sexuality and erotic energy more purposefully.
- Embrace my sexual freedom and the frequency of the Goddess of Love.
- Become more proficient at sex magick, and commit to working with, circulating, and raising sexual energy in my body.

If none of these resonate, return to the tarot spread and journal questions earlier in this chapter for clarity and support in coming up with an intention that feels right.

Step 2: Schedule

Your intention is set, and now comes the planning. My suggestion is to schedule your devotional around the Moon, consulting the section around lunar magick for ideas (page 201). Try starting a devotional on the new Moon; an equinox; solstice; cross-quarter day; or a significant date like a birthday, anniversary, or holiday. If you are releasing something like shame and guilt, you may opt to start at the full Moon instead. You can also check out what sign the Sun and the Moon will be in and plan to begin when these placements are supportive to your intention.

During your devotional, you will be performing a daily ritual. It can be simple like lighting a candle or saying a prayer or involve meditating and divination as well. The point is that you commit to it *every day*; because of this, you need to be realistic about what you can dedicate yourself to and for how long.

If you've never done a devotional and don't have an established daily practice, start *with five to seven days*. If you know you can say yes to longer, align your devotional with the waxing Moon, beginning at the new Moon and ending it two weeks later on the full Moon. If you already have a daily practice, extend your devotional to at least a month, from new Moon to new Moon, or even longer.

The key here is radical self-honesty. It's better to commit to a week and be fastidious about it than to plan a devotional for a longer period but miss a bunch of days. Keep in mind that you can always extend your devotional if you feel like it wasn't long enough.

Step 3: Decide on your everyday ritual/working

Now that the timing and intention have been set, the real fun begins. This is when you ask yourself, *What sort of ritual can I commit to every day and so honor my intention? What sort of daily working feeds it?* Again, this can be simple. It's better to start small than to try and do something elaborate, get overwhelmed, and quit. *Start with one or two things each day*, adding as you feel comfortable and as it becomes a habit.

- Meditation
- Prayer
- Journaling
- Lighting a candle
- Leaving an offering
- Creating art as an offering
- Divining with tarot or oracle cards and journaling around the results
- Practicing sex magick and moving energy through your body
- Dancing, singing, or playing music
- Repeating an affirmation or mantra

Pick a couple things for every day, or make a schedule, planning one or two for a few days and then adding or switching to something else, and so on. Allow your intuition and intention to guide you, and remember that you can always adapt around your experience. As the unfolding of your intention becomes more apparent over time, your daily practice can evolve to reflect this.

Step 4: Decide how sacred sex and sex magick play a role

Because this is a book about sacred sex, of course I am inviting you to make it a central pillar of your devotional. Do you want to take a vow of celibacy during your devotional and work with sex magick as you close it as a way to build up and then release energy? Do you want to have a daily sex magick practice so you can work on directing that energy? Maybe you want to practice sex magick only on Fridays, the day ruled by the planet Venus, as you work with orgasm and sexual fluid as an offering to Goddess, or maybe you want to anoint talismans you're charging.

Step 5: Create an altar to your devotion and intention

Using the steps on pages 41–43, fashion an altar that will act as the focal point of your practice. This can be as simple as placing a photo and candle on your bedside table, or as complicated as creating an entire shrine correlated to your intention. The correspondences you use should be correlated to your intention, and you can add items like icons or photos of Goddess/es, sex toys, inspirational smut, crystals, candles, tarot or oracle cards, representations of the elements, and magickal tools. Make it beautiful.

Step 6 (optional): Name your devotional

Names and words hold power. This is one of the tenets of witchcraft. It's said you can't control a demon unless you know its name. Naming something infuses it with life, so I invite you to name your devotional. This can be related to your intention, like "Devotional to the Erotic Votary" or "Devotional to the Goddess of Love" or to another personal goal.

Step 7: Dedicate the devotional

You have an intention, a timeframe, an altar, a name, and a daily practice. Now it's time to begin. The dedication is like the opening ceremony of the Olympics—it marks the threshold. This ritual will be customized to your intention and practice, but here's an outline for inspiration:

- Set up the space.
- Perform banishings.
- Ground, center, and shield.
- Cast the circle.
- Cleanse + consecrate.
- Invite in the Goddess/es you're honoring, if this applies.
- Formally declare and dedicate your intention, and meditate on this.
- Pull cards, meditate, and journal.
- Practice sex magick.
- Thank and dismiss Goddess/es.
- Close the circle.
- Ground and close.
- Perform banishings.
- Leave offerings.

For your dedication of the devotional, you may say something like this:

I, [your name], *officially declare and dedicate this devotional* [name of the devotional]. *My intention with this devotional is* _____, *and I am committing myself to this work from today until* [the end date/lunation]. *I am committing to this devotional through daily ritual of* _____ *as a means of purifying and aligning myself with the vibration of sacred sex. This or something better for the highest good of all involved, as aligned with my True Will. And so it is.*

Step 8: Perform your daily ritual, and check in every day

Now that the devotional has begun, it's up to you—yes you—to uphold the commitments you made. Remember, you are living this devotional beyond your daily practice(s). Be immersed in your intention and a vessel for its energy. Check in with yourself, your Goddess if applicable, your intention, and your heart each and every day, recording your experiences in your grimoire.

Step 9: Close and reflect

When the time comes to close the devotional, after the intended length of time or longer, it's important that you also formalize the moment. Follow the same structure in step 7, except instead of declaring the opening of the working, announce the close. You may say something like this:

> *I,* [your name], *officially close this devotional to* [the name of the devotional]. *Through this period of* [number of days/weeks/month]. *I have committed myself to* _____ *and learned* _____. *I thank* [the Goddess/guides/ancestors/ higher sexual self] *for holding me and guiding me and allowing me to move through this journey of sacred sexuality. I officially declare this devotional done, and the working complete. So mote it be!*

When you're finished, leave offerings and meditate or journal around your experience. Know the effects may not be obvious right away (though they often are), so be patient. The working is working. And so it is.

SAMPLE DEVOTIONAL

Intention: To embody the current of the erotic votary, Temple Priestess, and sacred slut

Length of time: New Moon to new Moon

Daily commitments: Adorning myself in red and gold jewelry, conveying my sensuality and sexuality in day-to-day life

Days 1–7: Researching erotic votaries, 7–10 minutes of meditation (+ celibacy)

Days 8–14: 7–10 minutes of meditation, 5 minutes of prayer, journaling around what the sacred slut means to me (+ celibacy)

Days 15–21: At the full Moon, dedicate a candle. Light the candle, 5 minutes of prayer, affirmations, sex magick

Days 22–28: Light candle, 7 minutes of meditation, 5 minutes of prayer, affirmations, sex magick

First two weeks: Raise sexual energy with visualization, breath, and connection, but no sex magick

Last two weeks: Practice sex magick daily as a way to connect with the egregore of the erotic votary

Name: Devotional to the Sacred Slut

Altar items: Red roses, photos of Goddesses of Love, red candles, gold jewelry, crystal dildo, books of erotic poetry, condoms, lube, rose quartz, carnelian, perfume, a letter to erotic votaries of the past, jade yoni egg, gold butt plug with roses, vintage BDSM postcards

Dedication

I, [name], *officially declare the beginning of this devotional to the sacred slut. My intention for this is to become an erotic votary by becoming a vessel for the Goddess of Love and sharing this in all I do and with those I engage with sexually. My intention is to connect to the current of the Temple Priestesses of the ancient past. I am committing myself to this work from today's new Moon until the next new Moon through daily ritual of prayer, sex magick, meditation, and reflection. This or something better for the highest good of all involved and aligned with my True Will. And so it is!*

Closing

I, _____, *officially close this devotional to the sacred slut. Through this past lunar month, I have committed myself to embracing and sharing my sacred sexuality, and I have seen this as a way to channel and embody the Goddess of Love. I have learned about my erotic power, and how I can use this to deepen my relationship with myself and Goddess. I thank Goddess, my higher sexual self, and all the sacred sluts of the past, present, and future for assisting and guiding me in this working. I officially declare this devotional closed and this working complete. And so it is!*

CHAPTER 8

The Path of the Dark God/dess

Trigger warning/disclaimer: This chapter contains descriptions of BDSM that include consensual pain and bodily harm. Please feel free to skip this chapter and path if this is too much for your mental health.

Sacred sex comes in shades of opalescent, iridescent, and glowing white as much as it does in ravishing, depth-defying, ravenous black—and every shade in between. This can mean reiki-infused kisses in the early morning and pain-inducing bondage in the evening, and now we will turn to the latter. This flavor of sacred sex is called the Path of the Dark God/dess for a reason. This isn't a path of spiritual bypassing, or rejecting the "negative" and intense in favor of something soft, safe, and warm. On the contrary, the Path of the Dark God/dess wanders intentionally into the shadow to see what can be toyed with, taunted, teased, and transmuted. It is through this path that kink and BDSM (bondage/discipline/dominance/submission/sadism/masochism) turn into sacred S/M (sacred sadomasochism), a way of embracing the edge as a means to radical alterations of consciousness, love, expansion, and gnosis.

This is a journey of devotional deviance, on which transgression is in the name of something higher. The reason you're here, and what you get out of it, will be unique to you. You may work with kink as an offering to a Dark God/dess or as a way to truly know your sexual self. Maybe you were told this approach is evil or wrong, but you know you're meant to be here. Breaking a personal taboo is powerful. Or perhaps you want to experience intense altered states of consciousness through the body.

Although it is still considered transgressive by the mainstream, working with pain, altered states, and intense sensation has been a part of spiritual practice since the beginning of time. This path isn't for everyone—in fact, it's probably not for most people. But if you're curious, and if you're willing to do the work to ensure you have a safe experience, welcome. And if it turns out this path isn't meant for you, simply choose another and take what you learned about yourself with you.

Sacred kink is all about radical self-knowledge and self-inquiry. This is a path that asks you to know your desires and reminds you that your beliefs around yourself, and around what's "right" or "wrong," create your reality. Taboos are a way to protect society from perceived harm; transgression takes place when these taboos are broken, which, when done with spiritual purpose, releases energy. This alongside the fact that BDSM is an energy exchange, and you can see just *how much potential there is to charge spells, rituals, and workings through transgressive sexuality.* Pro Domme Sydney Jones says, "As much as kink is a very visual and visceral experience, it's a lot about energy exchange more than anything, which is what sex magick is about. . . . You have an aim, you want to go somewhere with it, so you have an intention that you are setting to create this type of energetic arch in the experience that goes through different sensations of arousal."

Making something sacred means incorporating reverence. When you engage with BDSM in a ritual context, you turn the already highly ritualized act into a magickal working. Whether you're using spanking to raise energy during sex magick, bondage to reach an altered state, or sensory deprivation to feel pleasure in a new way, there are as many ways to work with magickal kink as your perverted mind can come up with.

Your kinks (or anything that deviates from heterosexual missionary sex and that turns you on) and fetishes (anything that you need during sex to be satisfied) become correspondences to utilize during ritual. You can work with kink before performing sex magick through masturbation or partnered sex, or *as* the sex magick itself.

This chapter shows you how to begin this journey. But first let's talk about safety.

SAFETY ON THE PATH

Back in the day (ten+ years ago), many described their practice with kink using the acronym SSC, which stands for "safe, sane, and consensual." The thing is, it's hard to define "sane." What's sane to me, like poking myself with needles as part of a ritual or getting suspended in rope, may be insane to you. This language also adds stigma to an already stigmatized group and subculture. Long story short, SSC just doesn't cut it anymore.

Instead, it's all about "risk aware consensual kink," or RACK. The truth is that engaging with kink and BDSM is a risk during which you are putting your body and mind in potential danger. Knowing this is key; consenting to this is key; and if this scares you, maybe this isn't the path for you—and that's totally okay. But if want to continue, then RACK means informing yourself of the risks and dangers so you can best mitigate them. This chapter is only a *starting point* on this journey, and not the journey itself.

Practicing RACK means many things, including the following:

- Vetting your play partners, or those you engage in kink with, by talking to them about safety, talking to their past play partners, meeting with them in a vanilla (or nonkinky) setting, and trusting your gut around their vibes
- Learning about where bondage and impact can be done on the body safely, and where it can't
- Consenting to the fact that you may get hurt, or bruised, or have an unexpected reaction to something (like an anxiety attack when you're bound in rope)
- Ongoing negotiated consent with all partners
- Having a safe word for when you want your partner to stop, or using the red/yellow/green system for when you want something to stop right away (red), slow down and lighten up (yellow), or keep going (green)
- Getting STD and STI tested regularly, and practicing safe sex
- Knowing your desires, and communicating them clearly

If you're curious about kink but have never done more than a light spanking in bed (or not even!), educate yourself by reading books and taking classes from BDSM professionals. The world of BDSM is thick and deep and wide. It's a never-ending universe in which every sexual inclination can be indulged. But more than this, there's a level of safety that must be explored that's beyond the scope of this book. Many of the go-to books on BDSM are outdated and written by cishet white men, but they still have good safety information. Check out the "Resources" section at the back of this book for some recommendations of where to start.

Domina Dia Dynasty offers this astute reminder for all new devotees: "Be aware that there are safe and unsafe ways to play with BDSM and start slow. Like if you're doing candle magick and you'd like to use the wax on yourself or another body, test the wax play out by dripping a small bit onto a less sensitive part of the body (forearm or leg) and work slowly inward. . . . And if you're playing with rope, make sure you or your partner have some basic understanding of rope safety and have safety scissors handy."

Taking the time to educate yourself will also lead you into your desires. When you learn about something and you have a strong reaction to it—whether it's a "HELL YES!" or "WTF?"—take note. Often the things that elicit the most intense reaction are the ones you will find you love or want to explore more deeply. Taking the time to learn basic safety, like where on your body you can flog and spank and how to safely tie together limbs, will also make you feel powerful as fuck and confident in the way you show up to your ritual workings.

THE DARK GOD/DESS AS INITIATRIX

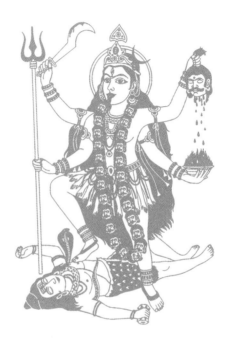

One of the ways you can begin connecting to this path is through the eyes and energy of a Dark Deity. A Dark God or Goddess, like Hades, Babalon, or Kali, are deities of the shadow. They linger in the liminal. They are often chthonic, subterranean, journeying to the depths of the underworld and taking their devotees with them. The Gods are beings with their own likes and dislikes, they have their preferences, they could be said to have their own shadows, and they all have the potential to be Dark God/desses. Yet there are some who own this title without doubt, which is what we will be exploring in this section.

The Dark Goddess of Love is the Divine Feminine embodied

through the lens of sacred subversion, through sexuality that's intense and vilified, and that feeds into an all-encompassing love—love that doesn't see good or evil, right or wrong, or whatever other binary we've been fed by society. It's a love that sees everything as love, even the dirtiest and most carnal depths. My own exploration of kink and BDSM is all dedicated to Babalon. BDSM acts as an instrument of gnosis, devotion, and strength for me because it's a way to push my edge as a masochist; reach altered states during ritual to commune with the Goddess, my guides, and myself; and to interlink intimately with my partners.

The archetype of the Dark Deity emerges in the Greek Hades/ Roman Pluto, King and God of the underworld, who acts as a guide to departed souls. Likewise, his Queen and Consort, the Greek Persephone/Roman Kore is also shepherd to the newly dead for the half the year she lives as Queen and Goddess of the Underworld. (She spends the other half as Queen of Spring.) Kink can be a dynamic portal for ego death, for pushing you to your farthest edge, which can bring soul-deep renewal. Call on Hades to guide you through the shadow and as a tool in helping to heal trauma and rewrite your stories, especially when done with a therapist or mental health professional, or with folks in the scene who are trauma-informed and willing to hold the space. Call upon Hades and Persephone for strength and guidance through this sacred exploration of the darkness and underworld within the self.

In this same vein, you work with a Goddess like the Sumerian Inanna or Akkadian Ishtar, who travel to the underworld as divinity only to be confronted with mortality and come back to Earth transformed. Inanna and Ishtar are associated with sex work and sexuality and may be called on to lead you through any experience that tears you apart and reforms you. Honor the Dark Goddess as you explore kink, no matter how dark or scary it may seem, because true transformation happens when you tend to these seeds of subversion. These Goddesses of Love and War show the duality and connection between sex and pain, between love and death, between darkness and the heart.

Another deity you may work with is Babalon, the Goddess brought forth by John Dee and Edward Kelly through Enochian Magick and later summoned through the magickal system of Aleister Crowley's Thelema. Babalon is a manifestation of the biblical Whore of Babylon, the Mother of Abominations and Mystery of Mysteries seen in the Book of Revelations. She accepts everything into her chalice of fornications, which represents her nondiscriminatory love and her ability to make love to all of the world. It is Babalon who births the Antichrist, or the messenger of a new aeon that destroys spiritual and religious life as we know it. To work with Babalon means sacrificing all you think and know about who you are. She appreciates and honors subversion and has a penchant for anyone embracing their own sexuality, especially if this includes sex work.

Last but not least, consider working with the Hindu Goddess Kali Ma. Kali is the destroyer, the abyss. Kali is the ego slayer, death but as a form of creation. Kali is a Goddess of radical acceptance, whose dark midnight blue skin is the color of the void. Kali invites you to face your depths with your eyes rolled back and your tongue lolled. She invites you into the shadow, for it is only in the darkness that liberation can occur. She is the Divine Mother who will protect her children fiercely, but only if they are willing to give up all of themselves for her.

THE DARK MOON AS
THE TIME OF THE DARK GOD/DESS

Just as rage or anger or sadness or pain all spiral, dance, shapeshift, and bend, the path of the Dark God/dess is also cyclical. This is the nature of magick, and the nature of the feminine, so working alongside the curves and crests of your depths is a big part of the unveiling of the shadow to see it as another part of *you*. Sometimes the frustration peaks, or the annoyance rages, or the envy spikes. Not attaching to this story is vital, and witnessing it so you can move consciously through it is everything. Kink in particular brings radical awareness to the present moment through intensity, pain, and conscious fear. Work with the Dark Moon to access this side of yourself because it is the moment before rebirth, the final stages of the lunar cycle when there's still no light on the Moon. After the Dark Moon, the cycle begins again.

The Dark Moon is the time of the abyss. It's the sensual, sexual, depraved, ecstatic heights of a peak experience, the moment when you feel both disconnected from this reality and one with everything. Yet more than that, the Dark Moon is an invitation to meet the Darkness within yourself. And let's get something straight: *darkness is not evil*. Just as you wouldn't call the night evil for the sun's absence, the darkness within yourself isn't either. Turn your attention to this aspect of yourself with curiosity. This is your moral, ethical self, your erotic essence that exists outside society's respectability. This is the crone, the ancient wisdom that lingers like a prehistoric fossil beneath the surface of the earth, waiting to be excavated.

The Dark Moon is a time when you can converse with your

perversions, fetishes, kinks, and fantasies. Try setting time around this lunar phase to begin your exploration. Watch new kinds of porn, or masturbate in a new way. Try a new sex toy with your partner, or explore a kind of sex you've been interested in but too nervous to try. Get your toes sucked! Tie yourself up! Eat ass! Get spanked or slapped! Try age play! There's nothing wrong with indulging in a fantasy if it's between two consenting adults. Allowing yourself to be curious and open, willing to try something new, is an incredible gift, and one you deserve to give yourself.

HERE ARE SOME WAYS TO WORK ALONGSIDE THE DARK MOON PHASE TO EMBRACE YOUR INNER DARK GOD/DESS:

- Research a Dark God or Goddess, and journal around what they mean to you and your sexuality. You may meditate or pray to this deity, or think about what embodying their energy would feel like and how you could do this. Consider creating an altar for them.

- Revisit your yes/no/maybe list and update accordingly. Look at the maybes and ask yourself which of these you feel comfortable exploring during the next Dark Moon.

- Watch new kinds of porn—the kinkier the better—and take note of how your body responds. If you feel a strong sense of disgust, take notes about what is triggering it.

- Try something new with your partner, or by yourself. Go on fetlife.com and explore the list of fetishes and kinks, have a conversation with your lover(s) about what you're curious about, and see if this is something you can safely explore.

- Write down your biggest sexual fantasy in as much detail as you can. You also can meditate on it and visualize it as if it were happening, and send this energy into the universe or to a Dark God/dess.

- Meditate in the darkness, and invite in your subversive erotic self. Show up with curiosity, and see who or what arrives. Who are they? How do they feel to you?

- Journal and meditate on your fears around sexuality and around exploring the taboo.

- Ground and shield yourself before you masturbate or have sex. Invite in the Dark Moon to act as a protective barrier, cleansing you of insecurities and fears.

- Spend time dancing under the Dark Moon, shaking, moaning, screaming, and being. Dedicate this expression to your subversion and darkness.

- Claim the title of pervert, freak, weirdo, kinkster, or whatever else you have resistance to. Use the Dark Moon, which only lasts for three days before the new Moon, to test out what this feels like. Record the results in your grimoire.

HOW TO INTEGRATE
KINK INTO SEX MAGICK

Sex magick has become a central pillar in my magickal and spiritual practice, and through my devotion to the (Dark) Goddess, so has kink. BDSM, when done correctly, is inherently ritualistic. Before you begin playing with someone, you negotiate and talk about all the things that you want and all the things that are off-limits. You talk about safe words and share any injuries, worries, or fears you may have, and you negotiate aftercare, or what sort of attention you'll both need after the scene is over. Aftercare can be a hug and water, it can be snuggling, it can be sex, or it can be a check-in text. You see if you have the same intention and share the right kind of energy, and only if this is a yes do you move on. The basics of responsible BDSM always follow this threefold process: negotiation, play, and aftercare. What does this structure remind you of? A ritual, obviously! First, you ground, shield, and set up the space, you move on to the ritual, and finally you close and ground again. BDSM naturally lends itself to being explored in a magickal setting. (That said, remember to first take the time to research and explore BDSM outside of a ritual setting. Get to know what BDSM feels like for you, what you like and what you don't, and bring that into your practice.)

In the following section, I share tips and tricks for incorporating different modalities of BDSM into your own practice, whether you're a top or bottom, submissive or Dominant, a masochist or sadist, single or not. In this context, kinks and fetishes take on literal correspondences based on the kinks themselves, any of the tools used, what the toys are made of, and what they do. Kinks and fetishes also

take on symbolic correspondences that represent what they do energetically, how they feel, and where they come from. For example,
hemp rope is literally representative of the earth and body because it
is made of hemp and symbolically represents pain; bondage; and being tied, bound to, or committed to something. This is by no means
a definitive list. There are more kinks in the world than you or I can
begin to imagine. Start here, however, and you will be guided in
finding new ways to integrate the worlds of kink and sacred sex.

BDSM will more than likely bring out some unexpected feelings.
Pam Shaffer, a kink-affirming licensed marriage and family psychotherapist (and Aquarius queen) notes, "When you are embarking on
a journey of sexual exploration, remember to approach your experience and yourself with kindness, curiosity, and patience. You might
discover things about yourself that surprise you or that make you feel
ashamed depending on the stories you have collected throughout
your life. Be curious about where your narratives and desires come
from," she tells me. "You can approach them without judgment in
order to choose which ones resonate for you and which ones you want
to discard. Be equally curious about shame or resistance, as it will
likely come up when you are challenging normative narratives. All
of your feelings are important information that can help you really
tune into what it is you desire and why."

Let's get started.

SIGILS AND EMBLEMS

One of the easiest ways to turn a scene or kinky moment into a ritual
is by creating a sigil or seal for an intention and then visualizing it and
sending it energy as you play. This can work even outside of a ritual
context when you're playing with nonmagickal partners. You can

create a sigil for a one-time intention or a seal to represent something more long term, visualizing this over a longer period of time. For example, you could compose a seal that represents your devotion to the Goddess Inanna, visualizing and sending it energy whenever you play, knowing that it is going to her as an offering. Dedicate this seal in a ritual setting in a way that makes sense for your practice, using the outline at the end of this chapter for inspiration. You can do this same thing with a sigil for a specific intention that you use only once, like if you're looking to draw in a certain amount of money or to find a new apartment within a set amount of time. Your intention can be mundane, too. It's just another way to support your desires, and the sacredness comes with the reverence for the act. It doesn't make you any less of a sex witch if you're getting spanked to raise energy for a new job, community, or whatever else you want or need.

BONDAGE

Bondage—which can include ropes, cuffs, plastic wrap, tape, and anything that binds the body and limbs—is a powerful way to reach altered states, especially when aided by breath work. Tying knots is meditative and relaxing, and if you're a rope top, this can be a way to get into a flow state and intensely present. If you're a bottom, bondage forces you to surrender and give up control, especially when paired with pain as in rope bondage suspension. Bondage can represent a contract or commitment that you are energetically binding or tying yourself to, and it can also represent the breaking free of patterns and energetic cords as the bondage comes untied or is taken off. If you work with cord or knot magick, rope bondage is a way to make this an embodied and physical practice, and because there are more resources than ever on how to tie properly and safely (like shibaristudy.com), learning is easier than ever. Practicing a sex magick ritual in bondage and then having sex or masturbating while still in bondage can fundamentally change the experience and give physical presence to your intention.

TEMPERATURE PLAY

Your senses are the gateways to magickal exploration. Working with sight, sound, touch, smell, and taste in a ritual setting invites a holistic experience that can bring you to new levels of altered states, especially when you integrate kink as well. For example, temperature play means bringing in the elements of fire or water. By charging and carving a body-safe candle and then using it to drip wax on yourself or your partner(s), you're taking candle magick to a new level. Drip the wax on the body in a specific sign, sigil, or emblem for more power, or on different energy centers or channels to activate these points. Slather on baby oil, or cover your skin with plastic wrap before wax play for easy cleanup. Wax play represents the energy of fire, sexuality, creativity, and will and draws in the erotic, the sexual, or the fierce and Divine Feminine. A working on owning your sexual power would benefit greatly from wax play done with an orange candle dripping over the sacral chakra or sexual center.

Or you could use ice to melt an intention into the body, like one for sexual healing. Use ice to trace the sigils, words, symbols, or emblems you want to be absorbed into the body, or over specific energy centers or channels, as you visualize healing energy being soaked into the flesh. You can work with ice cubes as a way to honor a Goddess like Venus or a God like Poseidon, or trace healing words onto a bottom's flesh as a blessing and cleansing. Alternate between wax and ice for a real mindfuck.

SENSORY DEPRIVATION

Sensory deprivation is a way of exploring the body and/or inciting fear through the obscuration of specific senses. This is a great way to attune the psychic senses—for example, blindfolds can turn the gaze inward toward self-discovery and lead to intensified psychic senses like clairaudience, or hearing psychic messages. Blindfolding in a ritual setting can mean an initiation through a dark night of the soul. The removal of a blindfold then represents a return to illumination or a rebirth after a period of darkness. Work with earplugs to represent listening to an inner voice or a deity or to force yourself or a bottom to surrender, all while inviting in psychic information. Gags likewise activate the energy center at the throat and prime you to receive wisdom through listening rather than talking. Because gags can be humiliating, they can also help you enter an altered state quickly, inviting in a new way of engaging with sacred sex. Practitioners who want to explore kink on their own can use blindfolds and gags for solo sex magick.

IMPACT

Impact play includes spanking; flogging; or using crops, paddles, leather straps, and hair brushes. When in doubt, spank it out, sticking to the lower half of the butt, and as always *be sure you're not hitting someone's tailbone*. (The top can place their hand over it as they give impact to help avoid this.) Pain is another way to reach altered states, and impact in particular is, too, especially in a ritual context when paired with rhythm and breath. Using your breath to match the impact is a heady practice.

Recite an affirmation or mantra as you give or receive impact, pray or visualize a sigil and send energy to it, focus on an intention like overcoming fear of your sexual essence, or simply be present and breathe into the pain to raise energy for the sex magick to follow.

CLOTHESPINS AND NIPPLE CLAMPS

Clothespins and nipple clamps are both good ways of exploring mystic masochism and intentional bottoming, whether solo or partnered. Clothespins are accessible, they're cheap, and they work. Because you can place many clothespins across a large surface area of the body by pinching them on skin, it can get you into an altered state really fast. (Keep in mind that the longer they're kept on the skin, the more they hurt when they are removed.) Arrange them in a specific shape like a sigil, symbol, Hebrew letter, or whatever else. Paint or buy clothespins in a specific color, or paint your sigils or symbols on the wood. Clipping them on specific energy centers like the nipples or genitals can bring awareness and energy to these places to charge a ritual or spell. Nipple clamps activate and awaken the energy of the heart center and/ or the Great Mother through the breasts. They bring intensity and pain to an experience, and meditating with nipple clamps (especially when paired with a ball gag and a chest harness) is one of my favorite ways to dive deep into altered states of consciousness. Keep clothespins or clamps on for no more than ten to fifteen minutes at a time.

TABOO

Exploring personal taboos and transgressing them with a magickal intention is one of the ways you can walk the Path of the Dark God/ dess. Likewise, working with taboos through sacred S/M raises energy and breaks societal bondage and can be dedicated to a deity you're working with. Some common taboos to break are exploring anal play; working with menstrual blood, vaginal fluid, and semen; or embracing a fetish.

Because the anus is connected to the root chakra, it can be worked with magickally to represent security, grounding, and personal fears. In this way, anal plugs, anal fingering, or even anal sex in a ritual can bring about security and grounding in the self or in the physical realm and release and dispel fears. This can be done in the name of Babalon, or a queer-associated God like Mercury. Menstrual blood can be used to paint or anoint talismans, grimoires, icons, or the body. It can be poured into a chalice with wine as an offering to a Dark Deity like Kali. It also can be consumed and imbibed as a drink and offering.

If there's something you feel a strong resistance to, examine it and engage with it as a way of exploring taboos during sacred S/M. This *will* get you into an altered state. Beyond that, it will raise energy and can become a ritual in its own right. Degradation; humiliation; objectification; and things like blood play (with someone you're fluid bonded to), piss play, or scat play can all become radical instruments.

DEDICATION

Another way to work with BDSM through ritual is via deity worship. You can do this by embodying deities and acting out scenes after invoking them into yourself. Think of how powerful it would be to do a solar working with Apollo invoked, especially if you drip wax in the sigil for the Sun over your heart using a yellow body-safe candle. Role-playing as God or Goddess or solo play with invocation isn't for everyone, so be sure to form a close connection with whatever deity you're exploring this with *before you bring in kink*.

If you are devoted to a deity with a predilection for kink, you may show your devotion through collaring yourself to them. The act of collaring is a ritual in which the Dominant places a collar on their submissive as a way to show that the submissive is owned or in service to the Dominant for as long as the collar is on. You don't have to use a literal collar for this—you can use whatever piece of clothing or jewelry you want—but the sentiment holds true. You can use a collar, a necklace, a piece of jewelry, or whatever you want to represent this commitment, formalizing it however you see fit. If you are engaged with an IRL power dynamic, you can dedicate this dynamic (or relationship) to a God or Goddess.

If you're a sex worker, you can dedicate your vocation to a deity or ask a deity to be your patron and protectress. As patrons of sex workers, Goddesses like Babalon, Venus, Aphrodite, Astarte, Inanna, and Ishtar are especially aligned with this.

KINKY SEX AS UNVEILING AND INTEGRATING THE SHADOW

Sacred sex is shadow work. When engaged with as a sanctified act, when honored with intention, sex has the potential to heal, transform, and allow new means of sensual expression. The Western world generally vilifies sex outside of a narrow prescription, which you've more than likely internalized. This is even more true for those who come forward with their history of sexual abuse or assault, especially for sex workers who have experienced assault or trauma, and in particular trans sex workers and/or sex workers of color. Being kinky adds another layer to this because BDSM was considered a mental illness in the *Diagnostic and Statistical Manual of Mental Disorders* until 2010.

Because of this, engaging in BDSM and sacred sex in general has deep potential to heal hidden wounds. Having sex on your own terms, no matter how vanilla or kinky, can be an act of alchemy. It can transmute old beliefs and boundaries by bringing awareness, presence, and intensity to sex in a safe setting. Therapist Pam Shaffer tells me, "Conscious sexuality and kink gives us the chance to use our creativity and agency to create pleasurable experiences for ourselves and our partners while increasing our capacity to communicate and process emotions as well. This all can lead to great feelings of acceptance and compassion for ourselves and other people which certainly is beneficial to everyone involved."

It's easy to reject the kinky parts of yourself, not only because society so desperately wants you to but also because they often live in the territory of your shadow. Wanting to be spanked or tied up or degraded or peed on, or wanting to explore age or incest or electro play, aren't acts deemed as "normal," so it's easy to compartmentalize, to reject this aspect of your sexual self. Through sacred sex and sacred S/M, you may safely and consensually try these things, heal and integrate this aspect of the self, and work with it as a source of power.

In my own exploration with kink, claiming the title of "submissive" has been incredibly healing, as this is not something I claim in my vanilla life. This has allowed me space to surrender to my desires and has been a source of strength because the submissive is the one who calls the shots in scenes. Fairy submother known as @askasub on social media and collared 24/7 submissive Lina Duna emphasizes this, explaining to me, "A Dom/sub dynamic is only possible as a consensual exchange of power between two equals. There's a common cultural misconception that submission is taken by force, but true submission is a gift the submissive chooses to bestow on a worthy partner." She adds, "Submission allows me access to a space where I get to experiment with vulnerability, both mental and physical. Knowing I have my own back like that, and that I can find my way into situations that meet my needs so precisely, gives me a somatic experience of trust within myself that I've only found to be attainable through this confluence of work and play."

Further, my realization that I enjoy pain has helped me recognize the ways I cause myself emotional pain. I have learned to note the situations in which I hurt myself subconsciously and change those patterns. When I recognize my masochistic tendencies coming out in my vanilla life, I can choose to engage with them differently and explore this aspect of myself in a more appropriate setting. In this same vein, consciously giving my power over to others and communicating my desires and boundaries in consensual settings has made me realize how I do this unintentionally in my day-to-day life. Because I know how much of a gift my submission is, I don't give it up to anyone anymore (unless they prove themselves worthy).

Kink gives you the chance to explore your erotic essence *without judgment*. As long as someone is exploring with another consenting adult (and not nonconsensually hurting anyone in the process), there's no problem. Your kinks won't be everyone else's, and vice versa. These differences can and should breed compassion and empathy, not separation and judgment.

THE DEVIL AS
DADDY OF DIVINE DEVIANCE

Unchained, unbridled, and unbothered, the Devil embodies a subversion of patriarchal ideals by reminding you that you get to embrace your humanity in any way you desire. The Devil is the fifteenth key of the tarot, corresponding to the zodiacal sign of Capricorn, one of the two zodiacal keys (alongside the Star/Aquarius) ruled by the planet Saturn. Like this planet, the Devil speaks of boundaries and beliefs that keep you tied to what others say is best for you. This is waking sleep, the illusion that each witch and magician must wake from so they can walk into consciousness.

In the classic Smith-Waite deck, the Devil appears eerily like the Lovers, except instead of standing in front of Archangel Raphael, the two figures stand in front of Baphomet. Baphomet, as personified by Éliphas Lévi with roots that may or may not trace back to the Knights Templar, represents the duality in all life on this plane of manifestation. Baphomet is a sigil, an energy, an egregore that embraces the idea of "as above, so below." Darkness and light must coexist, expansion and contraction must coexist, life and death must coexist, and so must pain and pleasure. Baphomet speaks of breaking this duality of other people's teaching, believing that everything is as it seems, and that there's a clear definition of good or bad and of wrong or right. Baphomet teaches us that *opposites are extremes of the same thing, existing at the ends of the same spectrum*, and that it's when you veer to any extreme that spiritual bondage occurs.

The figures have chains around their neck, but the chains are loose. They could be taken off, but there's no awareness of personal sovereignty, so they may as well be fitted tight. The Devil reminds you about unconscious beliefs you have that keep you tethered, impairing your growth and your evolution.

In the case of sacred sex, the Devil invites you to get a little freaky. What chains are binding you to old ways of being, and how can you subvert them, make it pervy, and break them in a ritual of orgasmic proportions? The Devil warns against swinging too far toward an extreme, whether this is indulgence or abstinence, and asks you to take a middle path. There's power in allowing old modes of being to decay and deteriorate (i.e., death) and instead delving into that which has been vilified. In short, the Devil is the Daddy of Divine Deviance.

JOURNAL QUESTIONS

As you know by now, conscientious sexuality requires introspection and exploration, even more so for kinky sex than vanilla sex. Not only do you have to know what you like, but voicing it with clarity and communicating boundaries becomes a necessity. Add a magickal element, and even more is at stake. Although this wildness is part of the fun, and although the unexpected is always an element of kink, you can show up more fully in your power if you do the inner work first. This is where journaling comes into play.

The following questions and tarot spread are meant to act as touchstones in your journey with the deviant and Divine Erotic. Use them to figure out what turns you on and what doesn't. Use them alongside other educational activities like going to classes and dungeons, watching porn, and reading books. If there are questions that don't resonate, skip them. Set up your space and yourself and then record your answers in your grimoire as a way to make them more sacred and so you can look back in a year and see how much you've grown.

- What does the Path of the Dark God/dess mean to me?
- What sexual taboos am I drawn to? Which scare me?
- What part of my sexuality and erotic self do I reject? Why do I have trouble accepting this part of myself?

- What desires do I want to experience but don't give myself permission to do so?
- How can I begin incorporating kink and BDSM into my sex magick practice? If I've done this, what have the results been like?
- What are the sexual and erotic experiences I am craving right now? How can I start to explore this, either solo or with partners?
- What does the Devil card inspire in me and in my practice with sacred S/M?
- What types of sensations and experiences do I crave or crave giving to others?
- What are my fetishes or kinks? Or what are the experiences and acts that turn me on the most?
- Do I feel more connected to dominance or submission? Switching? What does this mean to me?
- What deities am I devoted to that I can honor through kink? How can I create a dynamic that honors this devotion?
- What are my hard limits? What do they tell me of myself? What are my maybes? How can I explore these in intentional transgression?

A TAROT SPREAD FOR EMBRACING THE PATH OF THE DARK GOD/DESS

If you've been wanting a little bit of cosmic perspective while journeying through this path, welcome! Do I have a tarot spread for you! As you know by now, a recurring theme within the paradigm of sacred sex is releasing shame and guilt. This is because those feelings never completely go away, but, as the Lust tarot card of the Thoth deck demonstrates, they can be tamed, communed with, and even eroticized. Remember, they are feelings that point to what you consider transgressive, and transgression can be delicious. The tarot spread below is meant to give you a bird's-eye view of the path and how to dance through it.

Set up your space and get to it. And so it is!

Card 1: What message am I meant to receive on this path?

Card 2: How can I release and transmute shame around my desires?

Card 3: How can I more fully embrace and get off on these desires, kinks, and fetishes?

Card 4: Where can I turn for inspiration and support on this journey?

Card 5: How can I honor my subversive sexuality as a part of my magick?

AFFIRMATIONS

Remember when I said there's no space for kink-shaming in sacred sex? Well, guess what: that includes inner kink-shaming and inner slut-shaming, too. It takes time to release the expectations you have of yourself and your sexuality, no matter how deep-rooted they are, and this is intensified around any sort of kink or fetish you may have. The thing is, the more time you spend walking the Path of the Dark God/dess, the kinkier you will become. There are those who leave the lifestyle, as it's called, but for most people, kinkiness becomes a way of being and moving through the world. And like anything else, your relationship with it will be cyclical. There will be times when you let your freak flag fly high and others when you feel ashamed about being different or about trying things people make fun of.

Work with these affirmations when you feel the ghost of shame haunting you. Work with them when you want to remember how powerful you are. Work with them when you want to rewrite your narrative to be even more ecstatic, perverse, and transgressive. Work with them whenever you want to feel like a Dark God/dess. Don't you dare forget your power.

- I explore my sexuality in all ways that inspire me.
- My kinks, fetishes, and desires lead me deeper into my magick.
- I walk the Path of the Dark God/dess and embody my subversive sexuality.
- I honor my Divine Deviance as a path to growth and gnosis.
- I embrace the polarity of pain and pleasure.
- All my kinks and fetishes have space in my sex magick practice.
- I am a Dark God/dess of the Divine Erotic.
- I am allowed to be as perverse, as subversive, and as sexual as I want.
- I embrace my erotic desires, I embrace my sensual essence; I embrace my ever-evolving sexuality.
- I fuck my shadow into oblivion and then make love to what's left.
- My desires are worthy.

- I communicate my desires with passion, clarity, vulnerability, and depth.
- I have partners who are kinky as fuck, who I can trust, who communicate openly, and who help me explore sexually.
- Vulnerability is erotic.
- Trust is sexy as hell.
- I explore my erotic edge with pride and strength.
- I am compassionate to myself, and I honor my boundaries with gratitude and love.

A SACRED S/M RITUAL WITH THE DEVIL CARD FOR EMBODYING YOUR DIVINE DEVIANCE

You've unveiled your fetishes, come to peace with your desires, and excavated how kink and sacred sex interact. Maybe you've already incorporated S/M into your sex magick practice, and maybe not. Either way, this ritual will align sacred S/M with your spiritual practice by working with the Devil to release any baggage around your particular erotic expression. Sex magick is optional, and you can change your mind when you get to that step—although it's better to be prepared with toys and lube and then not use them than the other way around. Read this ritual first to get familiar with it and to tailor it to what makes sense for you.

What you need: Anything you want for your kink or fetish of choice (rope, a paddle, a wartenberg wheel, etc.), the Devil tarot card, your grimoire, sex toys or lube, and your sacred sex candle.

A note: You can work with a Dark Goddess instead of the Devil.

Instead of meditating with the card, meditate and invoke/evoke your deity of choice.

Step 1: Decide what kink or fetish you want to explore

Before you begin, think about what kink or fetish you want to explore, keeping in mind that it should be something that raises energy or gets you into an altered state of consciousness. If you're going to be performing this ritual with a partner or partners, negotiate the plan because each person will be exploring their own kink. You may work with a kink or fetish that excites each person involved, alongside the normal negotiations of what the boundaries are, who will be topping/bottoming, etc. Be sure to practice the kink *outside* of a ritual setting first so you know the safety protocols.

Whether you're partnered or solo, read back over this chapter to see what inspires you and what you feel comfortable exploring. If in doubt, consider spanking (yourself or someone else). It's easy, it's safe, it's versatile, and it's ace for raising energy.

Step 2: Decide on your intention

Now decide on your intention. Again, if you're doing this with a partner or partners, have this be part of the negotiation phase. Do you have the same intention? Does each person want to carry their own? Here are some examples that you may use or tailor to your liking.

MY INTENTION IS TO . . .

- Embody my Divine Deviance and subversive sexuality fully and completely.
- Embrace my kinks and fetishes as part of my magickal practice.

- Dive even further into transgression as an act of magick.
- Attract lovers and partners who help me engage with kink in a genuine, risk-aware, and magickal way.
- Dedicate myself to exploring sacred kink.
- Deepen my connection with my partner or partners through sacred kink.
- Release any fear stopping me from inhabiting my sexual self.
- Embrace the liberating force of the Devil as a conduit for my exploration of sacred kink.
- Dedicate a practice with sacred kink to a deity.

Step 3: Set the space
The intention is set, you know what kink(s) you're delving into, and who's investigating what. Now it's time to set up the ritual space. You may establish an altar for the Devil card, placing any black (for Saturn, the planetary ruler of the Devil card) or red (for lust, passion, and sex) candles here. Set up the space, be sure that everyone in the ritual has water, and, if you're exploring corporeal punishment or bondage, have some snacks like nuts or fruit around.

This is also when you get to make yourself feel like the Dark God/dess you are. Kink and BDSM are a fantasy. Part of this is glamour, and dressing the part, so adorn yourself in clothing, accessories, and talismans that align with your intention and are comfortable and appropriate for your kink of choice. Dress yourself as if you were dressing a deity, and care for yourself in this same way. You can wear something you consecrated by using the ritual on page 289. You *are* divine. You also may work with the bath spell on page 142 before you begin.

Step 4: Ground and center
Now that you have come to the circle as your fullest and most sacred self, perform any banishing rituals that are in your practice. Then move on to the grounding and shielding exercises as laid out on page 38.

Step 5: Meditate with the Devil card
Once you are centered, you (and your partner or partners) will be meditating with the Devil card in whatever way feels beneficial. You may visualize the Devil key as if it were in front of you, or you may gaze at it and breathe into its expression. You may visualize the figure of Baphomet in front of you—ask what they have in mind for you. You may imagine a body of light and project it into the Devil key, asking what the Devil and Baphomet have to share. Or you may visualize yourself as Baphomet or the Devil and see what this feels like. If you work with the Tree of Life, you can vibrate the letter Ayin, or the Divine names for Hod (Elohim Tzevaot) and Tiferet (YHVH eloah va-daat) as you meditate on the path of the Devil.

The intention of this step is to gain clarity around why you're doing this working, to connect with the liberating force of desire, and to access the freedom of the Devil.

Step 6: Declare your intention
After you have siphoned out all the wisdom and understanding you can from the Devil card, state your intention out loud. This declaration acts as a sacred signature, an act of commitment, a way of clarifying and dedicating your intention and the ritual. You may use the

following script, but really, say what's in your heart. If there are multiple people, each will take a turn to read their declaration out loud as the others hold space for it.

> *On this day, at this hour, I embody my sacred subversion and power. I declare my intention for this ritual to all the witnessing guides, ascended masters, and aspects of the Divine who work in 100 percent light. I dedicate myself to* [your intention] *on all planes, in all ways. This or something better for the highest good of all involved, as aligned with my True Will. And so the working has begun.*

Step 7: Work with your kink or fetish to raise energy or enter an altered state

Now comes the kinky fun. As you enjoy your kink, remember to come back to your intention and allow it to feel delicious and energetically emancipating. Also remember to breathe! If you are exploring this in a group setting or with a partner, picture the circuit of energy you're raising and sending back and forth, intensifying and expanding, together.

If you don't want to practice sex magick, raise and direct the energy for your desired intention now. When you feel like it's reaching its peak, send it out to the universe through the crown of your head, and through every inch of your body, like a beam of light so bright it can be seen from outer space. Stay in the afterglow as you feel your intention becoming reality.

Step 8 (optional): Sex magick to raise or send the energy

If you do want to delve into sex magick, now is the time. Whether you're doing this alone or with a partner, the idea is the same. If you were focused on reaching an altered state, use sex magick to go deeper, inviting in visionary experiences or psychic messages as they may. As you have sex or masturbate, enjoy the sensations and pleasure, noticing how it feels as compared to the kink you spent time with. As you have sex, move the energy up your spine to the crown of your head, until you feel like you're getting to climax. Then, send out this energy through the crown of your head. If you're doing this with a partner or partners and you don't all orgasm at the same time, each person will repeat this process of sending out energy into their intention as they come or get as close as possible. Stay in this afterglow of your intention, feeling it becoming reality.

Step 9: Close and ground
When you're done, declare that the ritual is finished, using the following as a guide, reading this together as a group if it pertains:

> *On this day and at this hour, I/we confirm and complete this raising of energy and power. Guided by the Divine Deviance of the Devil card, and the belief of sacred subversion as a worthwhile cause, I/we declare this working done, for the highest good of all involved. And so it is.*

Close using the steps outlined on page 39. Come back to your body, yourself, and your breath, feeling the sphere of protection dissolve back into you. Press your forehead or the crown of your head into the earth. Drink some water, eat some food, and come back to yourself. Practice whatever aftercare you negotiated on and then record this working in your grimoire, taking any notes of what happens in the days to come. And so it is.

CHAPTER 9

The Path of the Divine Embodied Masculine

I worship the Divine Feminine, which is something I often talk and write about. But what I don't share as publicly is that I also worship the Divine Masculine. In this age of patriarchy, when toxic masculinity is pretty much the only example we have in Western culture of what it means to be a man, worshipping, honoring, and embodying the masculine in all its expansiveness—and not in its most violent or harmful embodiment—is in and of itself taboo. Or at least weird. Our understanding of manhood is shaped by advertisements, true crime, and media that reinforces the notion that the tougher, the more macho, and the stronger, the better. No emotions, no feelings, and no tears, ever. This surface-level expression of masculinity leads to a confusion of authoritarian power with inner strength, and the outward forcefulness of male sexual expression at its most distorted emerges as sexual abuse and assault borne from a sense of ownership over someone else's body. The common story of masculinity is only one glamour, one expression, and one that has been manipulated and distorted. Patriarchy doesn't just hurt women, it hurts *everyone*.

To worship the Divine Masculine, the masculine in its sacred and archetypal form, is to hold up a middle finger to this narrow and ill-defined definition of manhood. Instead, it focuses on the power of the true masculine principle, the point before manifestation, the all-knowing potential and potency of life. But masculinity isn't evil or patriarchal. It's a projective and expansive energy that infuses the world with vitality and power. If the feminine is akin to the body and the earth, then the masculine is the animating principle that draws in life. Like the Divine Feminine, the Divine Masculine is personal. To embody your sexual totality means understanding that the spectrum of force and form, active and passive, expansive and contractive, mag-netizing and stabilizing, lunar and solar, hot and cold, negative and positive, and yin and yang, permeates all we do. Whereas the femi-nine may be experienced through the subtle body, through intuition and breath, the masculine is felt through the inner heat and passion that moves through you in moments of inspiration or arousal. Both take physical form, too, like when you're having sex and feel yourself shapeshifting into another dimension, or when you sense the presence of something greater than yourself.

To walk the Path of the Divine Masculine means rejecting the idea that the patriarchal formula is the only way to connect to mas-culinity, erotically and otherwise. This chapter will share examples of what it means to reject any received ideas of manhood and develop your own version instead. What matters is that space is given to the masculine *through* the feminine. This means experiencing manhood through the receptive, intuitive, and soft aspects of self, through the feelings of the heart and tenderness of the soul. When this is met with reverence, it dissolves into wisdom and strength. And when this same wisdom and strength is seen through the lens of the Divine Masculine, it turns into empathy and compassion that supports the world.

To reject the patriarchy means committing to another form of masculine expression. This is important to people who aren't men as well because you have all felt the pains and struggles of patriarchy and more than likely have emotional wounding from it. When you resist the idea that toxic masculinity is all there is, you begin to heal this hurt. You see another expression of manhood that is safe, accepting, and strong in a truer sense of the world. This allows space for trust and communication, which are vital for any of you who have sex with men. And for you, dear men, this means walking a solitary path that embodies the Divine through enacting your own purpose or True Will. This rejection also makes space for pleasure, for knowing your desires—*your* desires, not the ones that were ingrained into you—in a way that allows for rejection without anger or violence. This is difficult work, but it is incredibly worthy. The more you value the vulnerability and honesty that comes with living in a body, the more you give permission for others to do the same. Your sexual liberation is liberation for all.

The Divine Masculine is an energy of resilience and stability that comes from the self. It means claiming self-autonomy; it means listening to your own desires; it means holding compassion and creativity as core values; it means empathy, and listening when the people in your life tell you how they've been hurt by the patriarchy. It's the resilience to listen actively and then to do better.

The Path of the Divine Masculine invites you to embody the masculine as an expansive force that can create and transform worlds, not at anyone else's expense, but for the highest good of all. It asks you to stand in your power, to know yourself, to be grounded in your own virility and being with courage and reverence for the other. When you delve into sacred sex rooted in this approach, the masculine becomes embodied and gives space for the full expression of self. And that's true magick.

THE DIVINE MASCULINE
BEYOND THE EROTIC

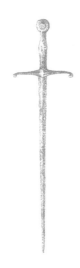

First let's discuss the Divine Masculine in a nonerotic space. It's important to remember that the expressions of the Divine Feminine and Divine Masculine are separate from gender and genitals. We live in a dualistic world, where things exist on a spectrum between two opposing poles—night and day, hot and cold, north and south, happy and sad. When I speak of the Divine Feminine and Divine Masculine, I am not speaking of what body someone is born with. I am speaking of frequencies that manifest in a range of ways, with these two energies on opposite ends of the same spectrum. Ryun Harrison, creator of the Abyss Tarot, a collaged homoerotic tarot deck, tells me in an interview that, "The Divine Masculine in summation is that spark of creation, the beginning, no pun intended, the seed of our inspiration, of our dreams, of the primordial before it's birthed." He adds, "People like to associate a gender binary to it, which I can see that we need that as humans to identify something that looks like us, but I think it's so much more about the energies behind those physical barriers. It's that very first spark or essence."

The Divine Masculine is the trigger for growth, expansion, creative expression, and erotic embodiment. Think of this when you decide to do something and commit to it, when you feel the first swirlings of passion and allow it to guide you into creation. It's the butterflies in your stomach before a kiss, a touch, a moment of sacred fucking. Rid of preconceived notions, this masculine presence can be a gateway to the numinous expression of the Divine Masculine, something bigger than the self. Just as the Divine Feminine or Goddess energy is that of immanence, the earth, and the wisdom of the body, the Divine Masculine manifests as the spark that ignites sacredness in everything.

Although I feel more naturally attuned to the Divine Feminine, I recognize that my discipline, my creative power, and my ability to infuse my erotic essence into all I do as aspects of the Divine Masculine. In my nonerotic life, this looks like my ability to work for myself and schedule my life so I can write books and teach about witchcraft, Goddesses, and the Divine Erotic full-time. The Divine Masculine shows up as my discipline and commitments: my nonnegotiable daily meditation practice, my commitment to being vegetarian, even the way I shave my head. The way I relate to the Divine

Masculine is as an unwavering strength and presence through the fluctuations and spirals of the Divine Feminine.

Taking time to recognize the Divine Masculine in your life and what it means to *you* can clarify how to bring it into your relationship with sacred sex. Redefining the masculine to serve you, as a means of support and positive reinforcement, can help you own your erotic worth. "When you think of [Divine] Masculine, what do you think and write down? And when you think about the [Divine] Feminine, what do you write down and think of that?" Harrison asks. "I think that gives you the two poles, the black and white of the polarity, because no one is just one extreme of the pole. We are all within the variants of gray."

The Divine Masculine means being assured in the self; it is not weary or questioned. It is known. The Divine Masculine is an evolved sense of power that comes from your core, *not from putting down others or the feminine, which is part of the conditioning so many of us have been led to.* Knowing yourself and being grounded is an expression of the Divine Masculine. Erotically, it's from this place that you claim your desires, find presence in the moment, and express your truth. The Divine Masculine is in action when you take a moment to go inward, whether before sex or when an emotion like anger sets in, to witness whatever you're feeling and breathe into it before acting. When you're able to do this and still lean into the creativity necessary to transform the moment into one of sacred ritual, or even simply presence, then this is the Divine Embodied Masculine, the masculine brought forth with the body as a conduit.

INSPIRATION AND EXAMPLES OF THE DIVINE MASCULINE

Besides coming to your own conclusions, and definitions, about the Divine Masculine, find some examples that resonate with you. It's one thing to have a conceptual understanding; it's another thing to actually see it. (If you want some inspiration, look at the art of ancient Pompeii, where the phallus was an omen and symbol of luck and potency that was featured in frescos, statues, and icons in houses and worn as jewelry.) There are many, many lived examples of the Divine Masculine—many of which are not erotic at all—but for the sake of this book, I will be sharing some of my favorite men who embody the Divine Masculine without losing touch with their potent and alchemical sexuality. This is by no stretch of the imagination a complete list. It's just a starting point to get you thinking about which related qualities you want to embody.

If you are a man, you also may wish to look to unexpected examples for inspiration. Therapist Stefani Goerlich emphasizes the importance of having a range of what it means to be masculine. She tells me, "Read books written by female and nonbinary Dominants, for example, such as Midori, Sinclair Sexsmith, or Princess Kali. Seek out religious leaders across not only the gender spectrum, but a variety of religious traditions as well. Starhawk's writings on spirituality will differ wildly from Rachel Held Evans, who will differ again from Rabbi Jill Hammer or Pema Chodron. When men engage with perspectives that they would never encounter otherwise? They learn a new way of thinking about themselves and their own lives and sexualities as well."

List any examples that come to mind in your Sacred Sex Grimoire so you can go back to them when you need inspiration.

LIL NAS X:
BOLD, PROVOCATIVE, AND UNAPOLOGETIC IN EXPRESSION

Hands down one of the most important rappers of the past decade, Lil Nas X is a gay Black man with lavish style who's not afraid to piss off anyone with his unabashed sexuality, all while slinging certified bops. His style and his music are an ode to self-expression and to love in all its forms, and specifically a homoerotic love that is otherwise unseen on the world stage. Unafraid and unapologetic, Lil Nas X exemplifies the commitment to the self that the Divine Masculine is rooted in.

APOLLO:
RADIANCE AND POWER

Apollo, God of the Sun, prophecy, and healing, was one of the most widely revered Gods in the ancient Greco-Roman world. Apollo is a solar God, whose twin sister, Artemis (known as Diana to the Romans), takes up the mantle of being a lunar Goddess. Apollo has an array of attributes that represent the multifaceted nature of the Divine Masculine, including ruling the arts, archery, and the Sun and protecting cities and herds and flocks. Apollo also reigns over the Oracles of Delphi, whose prophecies and visions were regarded with the highest reverence. In this way, Apollo represents the Divine Masculine as expressed through the feminine, through the all-knowing intuition that manifests in the body.

PAN:
EARTHY HEDONISM

One of the enduring figures in paganism is Pan, or the goat-footed God of ancient Greece who represents unbridled sexuality as manifested through the potency of the earth. Pan is a God of nature and the forest, with a cunning sense of deviant sexuality that pierces all he does. Pan represents the densest and most animalistic erotic energy available, one that is expressed and nurtured through the natural world. This God of lust and the primal asks for surrender to the senses while teaching you how to connect to the animalistic within.

DIONYSUS/BACCHUS:
DIVINE AND FRENZIED ECSTASY

The Greek Dionysus, known as Bacchus to the Romans, is related to Pan but expresses his power in a different way. Dionysus is a God of ecstasy, wine, and divine madness whose cult embodied these notions through orgiastic rituals and feasts that resulted in sacred frenzy and altered states of consciousness. While Pan's sexuality is rooted in the Earth, Dionysus's is of the body and its latent sensual and sexual power.

GOMEZ ADDAMS:
THE ECCENTRIC ROMANTIC

Gomez Addams is the romantic gothic King. The patriarch of the fictional Addams clan, first penned as a cartoon by Charles Addams for *The New Yorker* in the 1930s, Gomez has been personified in print, television, and movies as the beloved husband of Morticia

Addams and father of Wednesday, Pugsley, and baby Addams. Go-mez flips on its head the idea of what the masculine looks like. Instead of being assertive, aggressive, and inflexible, he is romantic, tender, and an absolute hornball for his wife. He offers an example of the Divine Masculine that is tenderhearted and unabashed in seeing this as a source of power.

RAM DASS:
LOVING COMPASSION AND SELFLESS SERVICE

Ram Dass is one of the most important and beloved figures to emerge from the psychedelic era. Born Richard Alpert, Ram Dass was a Harvard psychologist whose experience with psychedelics in the 1960s changed his life forever. His love and compassion formed the heart of all his teachings, which included those on mindfulness, devotion, service, consciousness, and dying, and his book *Be Here Now* was a revolutionary tome in getting the Western world to connect with mysticism and the subtle realm.

OSCAR WILDE:
AESTHETIC AND LITERARY INDULGENCE

Oscar Wilde's iconic quote "to love oneself is the beginning of ro-mance" alone assures his place on this list. Wilde was a dandy, poet, and gay man who lived a life devoted to pleasure and self-expression amid the background noise of Victorian England. His work, including poetry, plays, and his only novel, the "immoral" *Picture of Dorian Gray*, demonstrates Wilde's exuberant and expressive aesthetic. He was arrested for "gross indecency" because of his sexual and romantic relationship with another man and imprisoned for two years.

THE TABOO ON SEMEN AND PLEASURE

All the men listed shattered one taboo or another and, thus, represent the Divine Masculine not only through their commitment to their own boundaries but also by breaking established boundaries for the causes they believe in. It doesn't matter what gender you are, if you are committed to the Path of the Divine Embodied Masculine, you must be comfortable with breaking the mold. Masculinity has been diminished to a tiny box, and in that patriarchal box, there is no room for emotions or pleasure. To reclaim and rewild the masculine means expressing the inner self with awareness and care, living from this place, and transmuting this awareness into creativity and action. It means finding a way to sustain oneself while immersed in the grounding pleasures of life. It means embracing taboos and meeting the soul through the body as another way of integrating the totality of the erotic (aka the "embodied" Divine Masculine!).

Many people consider the body the domain of the Divine Feminine, but the Divine Masculine is found here, too. The feminine or yang energy may be thought of as the movement, the sensation, the exploration, the dance of the body and subtle body, but the masculine is the bones, the structures, the power and strength that can kick, scream, hit, punch, and yell. To meet the Divine Masculine through the pleasure of the body means encountering it through the physical vessel and the flesh.

Pleasure can be found through expressing anger and rage in a healthy way (like screaming into a pillow, *not* punching a wall) and feeling the space that comes from this release. Pleasure can be found through intentional touch, through movements that exert force, and through the sensuality of sex and sexual liberation. Intentionally leaning into taboo is another way to strengthen this connection, or to fade the harsh delineation between the Divine Feminine and Divine Masculine. The Divine Masculine expands, enriches, enlivens, and magnetizes. This means breaking boundaries that have been accepted as the norm. It's often not until someone does something that seems impossible that we believe it's even possible, and then it's inevitable.

Barrier breaking and taboo exploration can also begin in the microcosmic, in the body, with the self. And of course, this is a book about sacred sex, so let's start with semen. Although *taboo* may not be quite the right word, it does hint at the fascination and repulsion that semen often brings.

In a magickal sense, any sexual fluid that's involved in a ritual working, whether it's vaginal ejaculate, cum, or menstrual blood, has been charged with that working vibration and intention. The cum that's ejaculated as a result of a sex magick ritual or sacred sex working is now consecrated and can be consumed or used to anoint or charge something.

By this point in your journey, you know to pay attention to your strong reactions, whether this is attraction or repulsion. If your partner cuming on your face freaks you out, or if your partner spitting your cum back into your mouth grosses you out, or if tasting your own cum seems too far out, my suggestion is to embrace this personal transgression as an act of magick that feeds the Divine Masculine within. By breaking these boundaries on these taboos and desires, you are affirming to the universe that there are no barriers between you and the universe. You are dissolving divisions holding you back from the next level of your power and existence.

THE EMPEROR
AS THE DIVINE EMBODIED MASCULINE

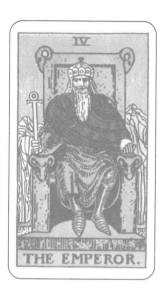

The tarot offers an archetypal reference for a range of erotic and eso-teric embodiments. It can encourage you to move through a tough situation or to show up more fully as yourself. And in this case, it is an invitation back into the masculine at its highest echelon. The Em-peror represents the duality of masculine energy that the world is facing right now. At its most encumbered state, the Emperor *is* pa-triarchy: the leader who serves his own ego, unconcerned and un-aware of the needs of his people. He is the resource-hogging billionaire who avoids taxes for his own gain, who lets the world starve because he can. He believes the only way to be a man—aka a worthwhile member of society—is through force and violence. The Emperor is harsh, unforgiving, and relentless in his quest to dominate and destroy. This is the warrior archetype at its most volatile and unstable, murdering the earth and its resources and subjecting women, children, and other oppressed classes to violence and catastrophe.

Yet at its most evolved, at its *core*, the Emperor is the Divine Embodied Masculine. When in balance with its complementary card, the Empress, he is a kind and compassionate king who serves the highest good of his people. He distributes resources fairly, he listens to his heart and his head, and he is confident in a power that he knows exists in everyone, not just him. The Emperor listens to his intuition actively and without fear. He doesn't feel threatened by emotions or love, and in fact, they are his guiding forces. He is the middle ground between the King of Peace and the King of War. He is both.

The Emperor is associated with the astrological sign of Aries, the Ram. Aries is a cardinal fire energy, meaning it burns away and transforms whatever it touches into a higher plane. It carries some of Fool's energy as it fearlessly moves the current forward and commences the zodiacal year. As the Emperor, Aries represents the heat, fire, and power necessary to live and lead from an aligned place. There is a burning and yearning in the Divine Masculine, whose boundary- and taboo-breaking power are most useful when directed with a clear-headed vision.

JOURNAL QUESTIONS

The path of the Divine Embodied Masculine, like any other, has its ups and downs. It also comes with its particular challenges, which you are of the utmost bravery for facing, beloved. To go against what the patriarchy instilled in you from the moment you were born is *big work*, and one way to do this is through the sword-wielding power of journaling. Journaling moves you deeper in untangling your views, acting as a road map in understanding what you believe and why. As you shed the beliefs that don't serve you, you make space for new ones. Journaling gives you the judgment-free opportunity to be honest and vulnerable about your desires while also marking your growth and evolution.

As always, follow the steps laid out in Chapter 1 to turn this process into a ritual as you wish. I see you. I love you. You got this.

- How do I define the Divine Masculine?
- How has this definition changed since before reading this chapter, if at all?
- How do I embody the Divine Masculine sexually? In my day-to-day life?
- How does reframing my definition of masculinity help me release the chains of patriarchy?
- How does working with my own expression and devotion of the Divine Masculine help this, if at all?
- What are my favorite examples of the Divine Embodied Masculine, and what do they teach me?

- How can expressing my inner Divine Masculine help me live, fuck, and enjoy life with more courage, creativity, and power?
- What old beliefs and stories around masculinity, both sexual and nonsexual, am I ready to leave behind?
- What new beliefs and stories around masculinity, both sexual and nonsexual, am I ready to embrace?
- How can this confidence be a driving force in my sex life?

A TAROT SPREAD FOR ACTIVATING THE DIVINE EMBODIED MASCULINE

Embracing the Divine Embodied Masculine can feel numinous and etheric. Without a clear road, it's up to each devotee to express it through their heart and body. Although I believe in the power of journaling and affirmations, I also know it can be difficult to work with something as noncorporeal as the Divine Masculine through language, and that's where the tarot comes in. Using the symbolic language of the cards, you can more easily influence and commune with the subconscious to bring the Divine Masculine into your being and life.

Set up yourself and your space. Grab your cards, and center yourself as you hold them and think of your question, whether it's what you need to know to erotically embody the Divine Masculine or something more specific. As you hold this intention in your mind's eye, shuffle your cards, pull, interpret, and record. Remember, you can use the tarot as inspiration for meditation, introspection, and ritual. Allow the cards to be your muse.

Card 1: How am I being called to awaken the Divine Masculine?

Card 2: How does this relate to my erotic self?

Card 3: How am I being asked to release old beliefs and stories about the Divine Masculine?

Card 4: How am I being asked to embrace new beliefs and stories about the Divine Masculine?

Card 5: How am I being supported sexually and spiritually by the universe while doing all of this?

AFFIRMATIONS

By now, you've burned away and banished the old beliefs you've had around masculinity. Filling that void with supportive beliefs and structures is the next step. The only thing you need to do now is the affirmations and trust that they will work. Besides creating new neural pathways, which leads to more supportive beliefs, attitudes, and stories, affirmations can help you recognize when those old stories come into play and give you the tools and agency to choose differently. Use the following statements to start this process, and write your own if you feel called.

- I am an embodied expression of the Divine Masculine.
- I embody the Divine Masculine.
- I embody the Erotic Divine Masculine.
- I express my inner Divine Masculine in a way that feels resonant for me.

- I release all old stories and beliefs of what masculinity looks like.
- I embrace my erotic essence and express this grounded in strength, creativity, and power.
- I find the Divine Masculine through my heart, through my body, and through my sexual and creative expression.
- My strength is a gift.
- All my sexual expressions are sacred reflections of the Divine Masculine.
- I work with the Divine Masculine within me to transform, create, and evolve.
- I am grounded in truth and compassion, and I show up embodied in the Divine Masculine as I practice the ritual of sacred sex.
- My sacred sexuality is expansive, divine, and perfect, no matter who or how I love.
- I integrate the Divine Embodied Masculine and Divine Feminine within me with love and care.

A SPELL TO BANISH TOXIC MASCULINITY AND INVOKE THE EMBODIED AND EROTIC DIVINE MASCULINE

Let me just start off with the truth: *no single spell will help you banish toxic masculinity.* But magick *is* a catalyst, a way of changing the story and rewriting the energetic blueprint. This banishing spell acts as the portal to banish the toxic, patriarchal masculine. But if it is not done alongside real, tangible work, then it's useless. You must meet the universe halfway. And because toxic masculinity is so ingrained, you may have to come back to it multiple times. Each time will strip away a layer of beliefs to reveal more.

This spell is a bit different from the others in this book. To begin, it's for you to do solo, and that's because it's vital that it banishes your own beliefs around toxic masculinity and the patriarchy and no one else's. This is intensely personal work. It is also different because it will be done over the span of two weeks, beginning during the waning Moon, a few days after the full Moon, with the second part on the new Moon.

This spell works with sigils, fire, sex magick, and the Emperor tarot card. Through sigil creation, masturbation, visualization, and intention, all paired with real-life work, you will begin to shed the restrictions imposed by the patriarchy. You will be able to more fluidly, easily, and authentically embody what the Divine Masculine means *to you*. Not to your friend, not to your partner, not to society, *but to you*.

What you need: Paper, scissors, a pen, a pencil if you wish, the Emperor tarot card, a lighter or matches, something to burn your sigil in to collect the ashes (a fireproof bowl, a pot filled with water, a cauldron), any sex toys or lube, and your Sacred Sex Grimoire.

Before you begin, make two lists:
one of the traits that you identify with and feel are from
the patriarchy and embody the toxic masculine,
and one of the traits you wish to embody and express
as the erotic and Divine Embodied Masculine.
You may also reminisce and write these before or during ritual.

TO BANISH THE TOXIC
PATRIARCHAL MASCULINE WITHIN YOU

Begin on the waning Moon,
a few days after the full Moon.

Step 1: Set the space, and prepare yourself
You're ready to commit to banishing the toxic masculine within
you—hell, yeah! That's a huge task! Set up yourself and your space,
as outlined in Chapter 1.

Step 2: Ground and center, and set the intention
This is the time to perform any banishing or other rituals that are
in your practice. As you're ready, ground and shield, as laid out in
Chapter 1. After you breathe into your sphere of protection, invite in
any deities, angels, guides, energies, ancestors, or muses, and ask for
their guidance. Meditate on what it is exactly that you're trying to get
rid of. Think about what the patriarchy means to you and what toxic
masculinity means to you. Feel it in your body.

When you're ready, write a statement of intention. You may adapt
the following:

On this [day of the week, day of the month, month, year] *I stand
before the universe ready to shed that which no longer serves me. I
hereby banish the toxic masculinity within me and all the ways in
which the patriarchy has shaped how I express, embrace, and define the
masculine. Through this working, I hereby banish the hold toxic*

masculinity and the patriarchy have on me, so I may move forward, grounded in my truth, on all planes, in all ways. I declare that [Share your personal intention here.]. *This or something better for the highest good of all involved, as aligned with my True Will. So it is. The spell's begun.*

Step 3: Create your sigil

Write down your intention, and cross out all repeating letters as well as the vowels if you wish, and then layer the remaining letters until you get a shape or symbol that you like. Play around and remember that the less it looks like words or letters, the better. Draw it on a separate piece of paper, large enough so you have room on the back to write, and then draw a circle around the sigil and cut it out.

Once you have your sigil on one side of the circle, flip it over write down *all the traits that you feel like you've inherited from toxic masculinity and the patriarchy.* Be honest! No one else will see this list. You may meditate on this and write, or copy the list you brought into the ritual. Write as much as you feel called, and take a moment to contemplate when you're done.

Step 4: Sex magick

Keep your sigil somewhere you can see it. Breathe into your erotic essence as you touch yourself. As you masturbate, stay present in the moment, and as you get closer and closer to coming, connect with your intention of banishing the patriarchal influence within. As you climax, or get as close as possible, gaze at your sigil and feel yourself banishing these demons. You may wish to come on your sigil, infusing it with this energy. Breathe and stay in the afterglow, noticing how good it feels to rid yourself of the crushing weight and expectations of the patriarchy.

Step 5: Burn the sigil, and visualize or connect with the Emperor reversed

If you came on your sigil, allow it to dry. You also can do this part of the ritual the following day. Visualize the Emperor tarot card or set it reversed before you, seeing it reversed as the negative embodiment of the masculine. As you feel called, tear your sigil apart, feeling its intention being released into the world. Then light it on fire as you feel the power of the Emperor reversed being banished, as all binds and chains the patriarchy has on your expression of masculinity are burned away. Keep relighting pieces of the sigil until it's ash. Flush, bury, or throw out the ashes, feeling this banishing being sent out through the cosmos.

Step 6: Close

If you invited any deities, angels, guides, energies, ancestors, or muses into this space, now is the time to thank them for their love and support. Let them know the ritual is done, and they are dismissed. As you feel ready, you may declare the ritual complete, adapting the following:

> *On this* [day of the week, day of the month, month, year] *I stand before the universe, filled with gratitude at this working of banishing the toxic masculine. I have released the patriarchy from my psyche in all ways and forms, as well as its hold on how I express, embrace, and define the masculine. The working is finished, but the commitment continues. And so it is.*

Once you've formally declared this working finished, ground and close, using the instructions on page 39. You may press your forehead or the crown of your head into the ground as in child's pose, sending any excess energy back into the earth. Banish if you need to and then clap, stomp your feet, laugh, dance, eat, take a bath, or do whatever postritual care feels the most nourishing. Leave offerings for any deities or beings who supported you, and record whatever came up in your grimoire. And so it is!

Step 7: Commit to this work IRL, especially during the next two weeks

One last step: commit to your intention in your day-to-day life, especially during the next two weeks. Find a men's group to join (if you're a man), read books, take accountability for your wrongs, question your feelings about women if you notice they are tainted with misogyny, and question what it means to be "a man." Use this time to actively undo your conditioning, which acts as a physical counterpart to the energetic work of this spell. It's not easy, but I believe in you.

TO INVOKE AND EMBODY THE EROTIC DIVINE MASCULINE WITHIN YOU

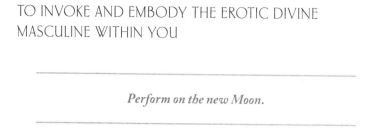

Perform on the new Moon.

Step 1: Set the space, and prepare yourself

You've banished the patriarchal masculine in the internal and external realms. Hell! YES! Now it's time to invoke the Erotic Divine Masculine that you want to embody. The first few steps of the ritual are the same.

Step 2: Ground, and set the intention

This time, however, your intention is to invoke and embody the Divine Masculine and the qualities in this that speak to you. You may wish to think of this and journal what this means to you before you enter the ritual space, or you may wish to do so during the ritual.

> *On this* [day of the week, day of the month, month, year] *I stand before the universe ready to invoke, embrace, and embody a new vision of masculinity. On this new Moon day, I invoke the embodied erotic Divine Masculine into myself, on all planes and in all ways. I call on this life-affirming, expansive, creative, fertile, and solar energy within me, to give life to all my desires in a way that's aligned with my values and beliefs. Through this working, I enter a new era, as defined by a healthy and supportive expression of masculinity. I declare that* [Share your own personal intention here.]. *This or something better as aligned with my True Will, for the highest good of all involved. And so it is.*

Step 3: Form the sigil, and list the traits of the
Divine Embodied Masculine

You will be creating a sigil in the same way as in step 3 of the previous ritual, but this time make it for how you want to experience and feel into the Divine Masculine. Instead of banishing the patriarchy, you're *mani*festing a new relationship to the masculine.

Once you have your sigil, flip it over and write down all the traits of the Erotic Divine Masculine that you want to embody, embrace, invoke, and call in. This is the version of masculinity that you are committing to evolving toward. It will take time, but this is a huge and worthwhile first step. You may meditate on this first, or you can copy the list you brought into the ritual. Write as much as you feel called, and take a moment to sit in contemplation when you're done.

Step 4: Sex magick

Be sure you have your sigil in sight. Breathe into your erotic essence as you touch yourself. As you masturbate, stay present, and as you get closer and closer to coming, connect with the intention of embodying the Divine Masculine and stepping into your power in this way. As you climax, or get as close as possible, gaze at your sigil and feel yourself literally stepping into this new reality. You may wish to come on your sigil. Stay in the afterglow and relish how good it feels to be erotically connected to this sacred vision.

Step 5: Burn the sigil, and visualize or connect with the Emperor

If you came on your sigil, allow it to dry, or do this part the following day. Visualize the Emperor tarot card, seeing it shift from reversed to upright, or place the actual card before you. Feel yourself *as the Emperor*, stepping into your role as noble sovereign. Then tear your sigil apart, feeling your intention being released into the world as you do so. Then light it on fire as it initiates your journey into the Embodied and Erotic Divine Masculine. Keep relighting the sigil until it's all ash. Then flush it down the toilet, bury it, or throw it in the garbage, feeling your invocation being sent out through the cosmos.

Step 6: Close

After you've burned and flushed the sigil, it's time to close. If you invited any deities, angels, guides, energies, ancestors, or muses into the space, thank them for their love and let them know the ritual is complete and they're free to leave. Declare the working complete, using or adapting the following.

On this [day of the week, day of the month, month, year] *I stand before the universe, filled with gratitude at this working of embracing, and invoking the erotic Divine Embodied Masculine within me, so I may move through the world grounded and rooted in this energy. The working is finished, but the commitment continues. And so it is.*

Ground and close, using the instructions on page 39. You may press your forehead or the crown of your head into the ground, sending excess energy back into the earth. Then banish, clap, stomp your feet, dance, eat, or take a bath. Leave offerings on your altar for any deities or beings who supported you, and record whatever came up in your grimoire. And so it is!

Step 7: Commit to this work IRL

Again, bring this into your actual life. You will continue shedding patriarchal programming as you step into this new vision of masculinity. As you release old beliefs, replace them with new ones. Return to your list of what it means to be embodied in the Divine Masculine, and use the affirmations, practices, and journal questions in this chapter to support you. Come back to this ritual whenever you need to, and remember that this is the first step in a lifelong journey. I see you. I believe in you. You got this.

CHAPTER 10

The Path of Erotic Embodiment

As you know by now, sacred sex isn't a path separated from the flesh, nor one that rejects the wisdom and power of the body. Sacred sex prioritizes embodiment, or living fully in the vessel of the self. The Path of Erotic Embodiment is rooted in expression of the soul through the physicality of humanness. It is one of immanence, a view that asks you to see the Divine, the numinous, the cosmic *in everything* and, in this case, especially the corporeal. To see the sacredness in all life means allowing the pleasures of this dimension to meet you where you are. It means seeing life as a manifestation of love, creation, and sexual energy. Embodiment, in this way, can inspire you to let go of the old stories that are keeping you from embracing the ecstatic experience of a life lived fully.

One of those stories is the idea that beauty and adornment are useless, frivolous, and unnecessary. This narrative says that anyone who cares about what they look like and what they wear, especially if they're feminine, is probably shallow and dumb. Those of you who, like me, have grown up in the Western world know the penetrating misogyny against anything women do, enjoy, and craft. Yet beauty and adornment—or glamour, which is a way of transforming something by veiling it—have the potential to be sacred. Beauty *is* the language of the Goddess, of the cosmos, and it can lead you to a state of Divine veneration, as anyone who has seen a lover embodied in their beauty knows. Beauty leads us to devotion, to adoration, to an expansive love. Beauty is also an aspect of fantasy, and fantasy is an important aspect of both magick and sex. In fact, glamour and fantasy go hand in hand, as the first garments most likely weren't to protect ancient peoples from the forces of nature, but to distinguish their roles in ritual and ceremony.

Magick transforms you from the inside out, and glamour transforms you from the outside in. Together, you have a holistic means of true evolution. To adorn yourself as a means of accessing your erotic essence and potential is real work. This doesn't mean you have to spend a ton of money, or any money, to link your inner world with your outer appearance. Sex happens through the body, so why not treat the body as a living temple to sex?

In the realm of sacred sex, glamour and erotic embodiment are paths to pleasure and to worshipping the body. To find the holiness of the flesh through breath, movement, and adornment draws the cosmos *into you*. Each touch or kiss, each fuck, becomes a prayer and testament to the Goddess, God, cosmos, universe, spirit, source. When you put on perfume, or drape yourself in gold, or dance before a lover—whether that lover is the other or the self—you are embodying your power and rooting yourself in the bliss of the body.

EROTIC EMBODIMENT AS GLAMOUR

Glamour plays a guiding force in my own relationship with the Divine Erotic. It is through my personal sexual expression, through adorning myself as Goddess of Love and Lust, that I am able to channel my sexual power into creative energy, devotion, and love. By honoring my body as a reflection of my soul, I form a union with the self. This is as much about the collars and slutty outfits I wear as it is about the dances and devotionals I perform for the Goddesses of Sex. It's as much about the collaging myself as an erotic oracle as it is about giving myself breast massages and dry brushing as forms of self-worship. Embodiment may start with glamour, red lipstick, and gold, but that's just the beginning. The body is the vehicle that allows me to honor my sexual self.

Work with the following list to inspire your journey with erotic embodiment, adding what resonates in your Sacred Sex Grimoire:

- Wear red lipstick. Everyone of any gender looks good in red lipstick.

- Wear a certain color, like red for lust, pink for love, or green for Venusian energy, to channel the energy of sacred sex through the body.

- Find the beauty in the ugly, in the decay, in the darkest crevices of what it means to be living in a human body. Allow all experiences of the flesh to guide you back into the holiness of humanness.

- Adorn yourself in layers of gold or copper, the metal of the Goddess of Love. The more, the better. Use the ritual in the next section to consecrate your jewelry as talismans of sacred sex.

- Dance, move, shake, scream, and cry. Call forth your most feral, primal, wild, erotic self. No judgment or shame allowed. Put on music or drums and move, allowing your breath and voice to guide you. Choose an animal—a lion, leopard, serpent, or wolf—to inspire you into becoming this beast. Notice how this affects your sexual expression and energy in your body. Use its print, colors, and correspondences in your glamour.

- Dress in something that makes you feel erotic. It can be lace, denim, latex, leather, spandex, or vinyl. It can be black, white, red, camel, cheetah, leopard, or sheer. What it is doesn't matter. What does matter is how you feel. If you learn that dressing in an erotic fashion isn't your thing, honor that. If you learn it's a quick way to connect with the Divine Erotic, honor that. Move forward grounded in this wisdom and knowledge.

- Create an erotic alter (or altar) ego to feed into your creative sexual expression. Be inspired by your favorite movie stars, characters, artists, and models, as well as tarot cards, deities, animals, and flowers. Make a vision board and a new name and backstory for this erotic persona. Use glamour to step into it. Practice sex magick as this version of yourself, and notice how it feels and what shifts.

- Define what being a Sex God/dess means to you, and write a mythology. Then express it. If you were a Sex God/dess, how would devotees pray to you? What kind of offerings would they leave? What sort of liturgy would they recite? What would your creation myths be? How would devotees adorn your icons and sacred art?

A RITUAL FOR CLEANSING, CONSECRATING, AND DEDICATING CLOTHING AND ACCESSORIES FOR SACRED SEX

The following is a working to dedicate items to wear during sacred sex. This can be a slip, a harness, a white ribbed tank top, a piece of jewelry, or perfume. This is a spell of glamour, so its focus is something you place on the body. You will cleanse that item of all energies with water, consecrate it with fire and sacred smoke, and finally, infuse it with intention using charged sexual fluids. Think: red lipstick for sex appeal, a leather harness for your inner daddy, perfume to invoke the energy of the Goddess of Love, etc.

What you need: The item you'll be dedicating, water (tap or filtered water, Moon water, rose water, Florida water, or holy water), sacred herbs (lavender, pine, cedar, sweet grass, myrrh, or frankincense), a lighter or matches, a bowl or cauldron, and sex toys or lube.

Step 1: Pick your adornment and your intention
Think of your accessories, clothing, and beauty items as correspondences. How does the item make you feel? What does it help you

embody? Consider these questions as you pick your item and set your intention.

Step 2: Gather the supplies, and set up the space
You know the drill. Follow the instructions in Chapter 1 to set up your space.

Step 3: Ground and center
Use the steps in Chapter 1 to ground and center. Feel in your body the energy you're calling forth. If your intention is to charge a leather harness with daddy energy, summon and call forth your inner daddy. Stay here until you feel your body buzzing with intention and energy.

Step 4: Cleanse
Once you've raised the energy in your body, cleanse your item with water, releasing any energies that don't support your intention. As you tap or sprinkle water onto your item, say:

Through the realm of the Divine Erotic, I cleanse this [item] *of all that is not in service. Only that which is aligned with my sacred sexual expression may remain. I clear this of any negative and un-necessary energy that doesn't vibrate with 100 percent Divine light on all planes and in all ways.*

Feel white light pouring from the heavens, through your body, into the item. Visualize the water washing away anything not aligned with the spell.

Step 5: Consecrate

Repeat this process but with fire and smoke. Light your herbs and blow them out so they smoke. Pass your item through the smoke, visualizing it as cleansing white light, and say:

> *Through the realm of the Divine Erotic, I consecrate this* [item] *in the name of sexual embodiment. May this item serve as a divine vessel of charged power, imbuing me in all ways and all planes with its sacred vibration. May this help me connect to my truest erotic potential, in all planes, and all ways.*

Feel white light pouring from the heavens, through your body, into the item. Visualize the smoke imbuing it with sacred sexual energy.

Step 6: Sex magick for sexual fluid

Note: you can skip this step if you don't feel comfortable with it! You will be doing sex magick to charge your item, which you will then anoint with bodily fluid (which can be sexual, spit, blood, or sweat). As you masturbate or have sex, feel yourself expressed in the energy you want this item to cultivate. Feel this as truth, and as you climax, or get as close as possible, send the energy through the crown of your head into the cosmos. Continue this visualization in the afterglow as you fully inhabit this space and truth.

Step 7: Anoint

Feel the power you raised as golden light coursing through your body. As you're ready, take your sexual fluids, whether vaginal secretions, semen, sweat, blood, or spit, and anoint your item (it can be on the inside or tag) and say the following:

Through the realm of the Divine Erotic, I imbue this [item] *with sacred sexual intention. May this serve me in expressing* [your intention] *on all planes and in all ways, always. May it help me channel my most divine and intoxicating sexuality and call forth the erotic powers within me effortlessly. I now affirm this item sexually and magickally charged, as aligned with my True Will for the highest good of all involved. And so it is!*

Feel the divine energy of the universe moving through you, into this item. Feel it as a portal to sacred sex through the flesh.

Step 8: Close the ritual, and work with the item

Find a comfortable seat, and turn your gaze inward, charged item in hand or nearby. Close your eyes, and notice how you feel. When you feel called to close and ground, do so.

You may wear the item(s) you consecrated only in a formal ritual setting, or to integrate your erotic power whenever the hell you wish, whether this is on a date, at a sex party, out dancing, or when you want to be that bitch running errands or hanging out in the coffee shop. Just don't forget that these are sacred items and should be cared for and treated as such. Place your jewelry in color-appropriate velvet pouches, or keep them on your altar; display your garments; put the perfume on a beautiful vanity; or hang up your lingerie on velvet hangers. Allow yourself to enjoy the sensuality of this experience. And so it is.

SEX GLAMOUR ICONS AS MUSE

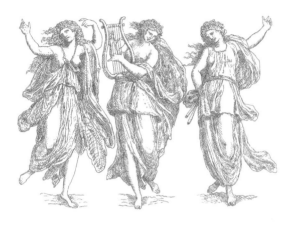

One way to unveil your own erotic alchemical glamour is through recognizing who inspires you to tap into your sexual essence on a physical level. Who are your muses who work with fashion and beauty as a means of expressing their inner worlds? Being aware of what does and doesn't resonate in this way is an important *and fun* starting point in creating a personal style that aligns with your sexual values, interests, and beliefs. The most influential style icons in my own life share the thread of sexual expression: Morticia Addams, Poison Ivy of the Cramps, Vivienne Westwood, Catwoman, and Elvira, to name a few. Creating your own list or vision board of fashion inspiration, and journaling around *what exactly* inspires you, can help you understand your own erotic magick more clearly—or at the very least, give you great references for outfit ideas.

Here are a few examples of femme fatales, Goddesses, and muses who work with sexuality and sacred perversion to craft a glamour all their own. Hopefully, they will help you do the same.

Goddesses of Love and Lust: The Goddesses of Love and Lust are wonderful muses to work with, conjure, and honor. Not only will doing so invite more love and sex into your life (because you *become* the love and sex you desire), but she also can help you express beauty in a new way.

Turn to art and myth for aesthetic inspiration. Venus and Aphrodite, Goddesses of beauty, sex, love, and desire, are often seen naked, with nothing but golden hair draped around their shoulders. Venus Aphrodite is also known for her sacred girdle, which makes anyone who gazes upon her fall in love and was inherited from her predecessors, Inanna or Ishtar. You can consecrate your own using the previous ritual.

Prince: What can you write about a fashion and music icon, muse, and divine pervert whose vision and voice are as timeless and recognizable as his favorite color and the symbol he once used to replace his name? With his love of purple, his skintight outfits, and his undeniable eroticism, Prince was a legend and divine sexual royalty for a reason. May his legacy, his power, his lust, and his incredible eye for fashion inspire your own journey of liberated sexuality and sexual expression.

David Bowie: One of the most striking acts of magick conjured by David Bowie in his many incarnations is the inability to fit him into a single box. Bowie used magick, ritual, glamour, and self-creating (and self-sustaining) images and visuals to manifest an unsurpassed erotic archetype. May he act as a guide in embracing every part of who you are, sexually and creatively, as an ode to your soul and truest self.

Madonna: Madonna is more than just a pop star; she is an emblem of unsuppressed and unbridled feminine sexuality. She works with provocation, performance, and embodiment and is basically a Goddess of Sacred Subversion. Madonna uses her stage persona, her art, and her music to juxtapose the pure and the profane, the sacred and the taboo. Madonna assembles a potent erotic expression that you can call upon when you want to be reminded of the power inherent in the flesh.

THE PATH OF EROTIC EMBODIMENT AS MOVEMENT

One way you may experiment with this path is by focusing on moving your body rather than adorning it. Sex happens with the body, and movement practices like yoga asanas, dancing, and breath are other avenues to your erotic self. Even if your intention for yoga or dance is for greater self-awareness, this will lead you to a deeper understanding and connection with your sexuality as well.

Below, find some simple practices inspired by yoga, movement, and breath to help you along the Path of Erotic Embodiment.

1. Cat cow pose:

Find a comfortable place, preferably on a yoga mat, and get on all fours, hands shoulder-width apart and knees hip-width apart. Your spine should be long and straight. Inhale, and arch your spine and butt up to the ceiling, taking cow pose. Feel this stretch in your back and your hips, but be sure to listen to your body—don't overdo it! As you exhale, round your spine, and bring your head and hips down, like a cat hissing in the classic Halloween pose. Follow your breath, and move at your own pace, moving into cow pose as you inhale and cat pose as you exhale. As you inhale, pull the energy from your sexual center through the central channel of your body toward the crown chakra, and as you exhale, pull this energy down from the crown to the root chakra. Repeat this for at least two minutes, taking any notes of what came up in your Sacred Sex Grimoire.

2. Breath of fire with root lock:

In this exercise, you will be practicing a breath correlated to the element of fire and pairing it with an energy lock, or what's known as a bandha in the yogic tradition. In this case, you'll be working with the root lock, or mula bandha, to stop energy flow from moving down the body and out of the sexual organs. Practicing this lock can delay ejaculation and can help those with penises achieve semen retention, but it can be done with anyone of any anatomy. In those with vulvas, it can help intensify orgasms. To get familiar with what this feels like, pee and then stop the flow of urine. The root lock should activate this muscle and pull it up. For those of you with vulvas, this feels similar to doing a Kegel, except you draw up the energy and pelvic floor.

The breath used during mula bandha is related to the tattva of tejas. In the Hindu tradition, tattvas (which mean "reality" or "truth") take the form of elements, and that of tejas is the tattva of fire, which is represented by a red triangle against a green background. The breath is energizing and purifying and follows the path of an inverted triangle, meaning it's an inhalation, a holding of the breath, and an exhalation before beginning again.

Start with four seconds for each side of the triangle: inhale . . . hold . . . and exhale. Once you get comfortable, slow down your breath, holding all parts for equal amounts of time. Visualize and trace an upside-down triangle, starting at the root chakra, as you inhale and move up to one shoulder, then to the other as you hold the breath, and move from that shoulder back to the root chakra as you exhale.

While you hold the breath, you will perform the root lock or mula bandha. Breathe in for four counts, and as you hold for four counts, engage the muscle at the root of the sexual organs and pull up like you're stopping the flow of pee. Then, as you exhale for four counts, release. Do this for two minutes and then breathe normally, seeing how you feel. If you want to take this to the next level, practice this as you masturbate and then as you have sex. I love to work with this breath and bandha as I am meditating because it activates the erotic energy within me and allows me to direct it with ease and even reach altered states of consciousness.

3. Dance, shake, and scream it out:

Move, move, *move*. Move as if your erotic essence is guiding you. Breathe into your erotic center and then dance, shake, jab, scream, and growl as you unleash this energy. Feel into your body without judgment and without thinking about how you look or if you're doing it right. (Even if you can only move one part of your body or can't stand or move fluidly, your mind can still break past all expectations.) Move from different parts of your body, make sounds, and laugh. Get lost in the dance, movement, shaking, or thought of this. Come back to yourself over and over again. When the ritual feels complete, thank yourself and record anything that came up in your grimoire. This also is a fun activity to do with a partner because it requires an immense amount of vulnerability.

THE STAR:
THE GUIDE TO LIVING SENSUALITY

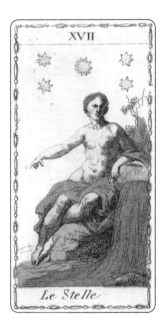

The Star may not seem like the obvious choice for a chapter on glamour and sexual self-expression because the Star is classically naked.

But she is also surrounded by stars in the sky, and she exudes a sense of divinely calm radiance. The Star may not be draped in vestments of beauty, but she *is* beauty and she is divine guidance that comes from living aligned with one's truth. The Star represents embodiment beyond any physical accruements.

The Star is the power that comes from unapologetically living in the flesh. Her erotic expression may start with her clothes, but even in her most naked and vulnerable state, the Star is nothing but totally grounded and confident. The Star tells you it's your right and destiny to feel safe and at home in who you are. It is your right to be expressed in whatever way feels delicious and fulfilling, whether that's through an excess of adornment or none at all. This key unlocks the magick of completely coming home as a brilliant spark within this universe.

As the tarot card for Aquarius, the Water Bearer, the Star embodies the ideal that grounding in your erotic truth and expressing yourself fully holds space and gives permission for others to do the same. Aquarius is the humanitarian, the trailblazer, and the star is this inner divine guidance that allows the energy of the fixed air sign of Aquarius to follow their own path with confidence. On the Path of Erotic Embodiment, the Star as Aquarius energy speaks of the freedom you give yourself and the world when aligned within your own power.

JOURNAL QUESTIONS

Journaling around embodiment can be particularly powerful because it is so hard to truly experience embodiment without the mind getting involved. Journaling lets you work with the mind to think, prod, analyze, and explore the body and its erotic potential. Then, when it comes to be practice rituals of adornment, adoration, and glamour, the mind has already done its thing and thought its thoughts, which leaves space for presence and feeling.

Write your answers in your Sacred Sex Grimoire, collage, brain map, doodle, free write; there is no wrong way to dive into these prompts.

- Where in my body do I feel the Divine Erotic? How does this feel in different parts of my body?
- What does embodiment mean to me? How is this a part of my sacred sex or sex magick practice?
- What activities and practices can I rely on to feel embodied and not just in my head?
- How does adorning, dressing, and decorating my being help me feel embodied in myself?
- Who are my role models and muses when it comes to erotic embodiment and sexual self-expression?
- What alter/altar egos can I uncover to find new facets of my erotic self?
- How do I feel and move through life when I am truly expressed in my power and sexuality? How can I consciously live from this place more fully?
- What items help me tap into my beauty, my glamour, my sexuality? How can I work with these in rituals of beauty and self-devotion?
- What does the Star card mean to me? How does it speak to me of erotic embodiment?
- How can dance, breath, movement, and other practices of embodiment help me find more compassion for where my body is, right here, right now?

- What can I wear to feel the most myself in my body and glamour?

A TAROT SPREAD FOR EROTIC EMBODIMENT

This tarot spread will help you work with all aspects of yourself as you dance along the path of erotic embodiment. It's here to provide perspective on how to work alongside your mind, alongside your spirit, and alongside your body. Instead of rejecting the mind in lieu of the body, this spread invites all aspects of who you are, and all aspects of your experience as a human being, into the divine world of the sacred sexual.

Before beginning, I strongly suggest exploring some kind of embodiment ritual, as it will help you feel this experience with more clarity. When you're ready, breathe as you ask your cards your question. This may be something specific around embodiment and sexual expression, or it may be something simple like, "How am I being called to show up embodied in my erotic energy right now?" Shuffle the cards as you hold this question in mind, cut the deck if it's in your practice, pull, interpret, and record. Meditate with whatever cards for which you want to further explore their energies, or try working with the cards as aesthetic and glamour inspiration. Allow these keys to be creative forces and muses in your erotic exploration. And so it is.

Card 1: How am I being called into erotic embodiment?
Card 2: How can I work alongside my mind to meet my true sexual self-expression?

Card 3: How can my creativity and muses play a part of this?

Card 4: How can I challenge myself creatively with this?

Card 5: What wisdom am I meant to take with me on this path?

AFFIRMATIONS

Yes, I know, I just told you that you can't think your way to embodiment. And while it may seem contrary to work with affirmations as a supplement to this, the truth is that to feel as embodied as possible, you need your mind on your side and not against it. This means affirming your strength, your power, your glamour, and your beauty. This means giving yourself pep talks before you dress the fuck up or show the fuck up through dance, movement, or any other form of ecstatic expression. Affirmations are an anchor when you're trying on different selves or exploring different parts of your heart. They could never replace an embodiment practice, or sacred sexual adornment, but they can give you the confidence to go after whatever creative vision you're holding in your third eye.

These affirmations are here to remind you that you have every right to live fully in your body, with all the magickal, mystical, painful, pleasurable, beautiful, and expansive energies that reside therein.

- I am embodied in my truest erotic expression.
- I walk the Path of Erotic Embodiment with confidence, purpose, and inspiration.
- My body is a vessel of the Divine.
- My body is a pathway to the erotic.
- I am an embodiment and expression of the Divine Erotic.

- I breathe into my being and feel the ecstasy of presence.
- I honor my body. I love my body. I trust my body.
- My sexuality leads me deeper into myself, my body, my purpose, and my heart.
- I express myself in a way that honors my fullest self.
- My sexual and creative self-expression are magickal and sacred as fuck.
- I follow the wisdom of the Star and honor the body as a gateway to the ecstatic erotic.
- I experience sacred sex through the flesh, embodied in my power.
- My body is my channel to the Divine Erotic. I honor it with love, compassion, and gratitude.

A GLAMOUR RITUAL
OF BODY AND FLESH
INSPIRED BY INANNA'S DESCENT

Embodiment begins with the flesh. It is the opening, a sacred gate into embodiment as a mode of living. This ritual is inspired by the descent of the Sumerian Goddess Inanna to the underworld, the oldest recorded myth, where she goes to witness the funeral of her sister Ereshkigal's husband, Gugalanna. But Ereshkigal, Inanna's twin sister, has other plans. As Inanna, Queen of Heaven and Earth, makes her way to her sister's domain, she is forced to remove an item of her clothing as she passes through each of the Seven Gates to the Underworld. Inanna arrives naked and mortal. Ereshkigal pierces Inanna and hangs her on a hook for three days and nights, like a piece of meat. Inanna is able to escape, thanks to her attendant Nin-shubur and Enki, the God of Wisdom. But Ereshkigal demands a return and sacrifice, so Inanna chooses her husband, Dumuzi, whom she finds sitting on her throne and not worried at all about his wife's sudden disappearance. Dumuzi ends up spending half the year in the underworld, and his sister spends the other six months there as his replacement.

Inanna comes back from the underworld transformed, integrated, and whole in a way only a dark night of the soul can initiate. Inanna has just gone through the Goddesses' Journey. It is only by stripping bare, releasing her ego attachments, and allowing herself to be in complete submission to the cosmos that she can make her way back up to the earth. She descends into the underworld as Queen of Heaven and Earth and returns as Queen of Heaven, Earth, and Underworld. This is a metaphor both for shadow work and transmuting darkness into power as much as it is for journeying into the subconscious and unconscious mind and bringing new aspects of the self to light.

The framework of this ritual is the stripping of garments to reveal your mortality. You will be choosing seven layers of items to represent seven parts of yourself and then ritually shedding these and blessing yourself in your fullest mortality and humility. Like the Star twinkling after the fall of the Tower, you will then step into yourself in your fullest erotic expression.

The seven items should represent, respectively: *the will, the ego, the mind/patterns, the sexual self, yearning for illumination, magick,* and *divinity.* Or choose seven items based on the planets or chakras, or seven aspects of yourself that are keeping you from embodying your erotic self. They can be a pair of earrings, necklaces, articles of clothing, shoes, lingerie, a hat, gloves, or a coat. This is where personal creativity and magick come in, as does your relationship with glamour and adornment. *By the time you remove every article of clothing, you should be completely naked.* If you don't feel comfortable with this, you may remain in something that still challenges your personal limits, like a slip or pair of boxers.

In the mythos, the following is what Inanna gave up at each gate:

1st gate: Her crown
2nd gate: Her lapis necklace
3rd gate: Her breast beads
4th gate: Her breastplate
5th gate: Her gold ring
6th gate: Her lapis measuring rod and line
7th gate: Her royal robe

What you need: Your Sacred Sex Grimoire, the Star tarot card, lube and/or a sex toy, and your sacred sex candle.

This ritual is meant for a single individual because glamour is incredibly personal, and this is a working of inner alchemy.

Step 1: Set up the space and self

This is an intense ritual, and I suggest taking a ritual bath either before or as aftercare. Either way, gather your supplies and figure out your seven items and what they represent. This is a ritual of glamour and embodiment, so dress the fuck up and make yourself feel like a damn God/dess. Take the time to ritualize this process as much as you wish and then set up the space.

Step 2: Get clear on the intention

Once your space is set, get clear on your intention. Then record what each of your seven chosen garments represent. This is a ritual of ego death, of transformation, and surrender. Afterward, you will have leaped into a portal of Divine Embodiment. You will have declared your aspiration to live in your body as an avatar of the Divine, even after being stripped of all your attachments, expectations, and ideas of self. This is a ritual of erotic embodiment, yes, but it's just as much of a ritual of death and rebirth. What aspects of yourself are you ready to release? It can be an old pattern and way of thinking about your body, it can be something literal like an attachment to an aesthetic, or it can be emotional like only feeling beautiful under certain circumstances. Get out your journal and write, perhaps also pulling a tarot or oracle card for each item you're going to be wearing.

Then, write a declaration of erotic embodiment. This will propel you into a new state of exploration. This is your declaration of being in a collaborative partnership with the universe. This is your declaration of a new, refined, evolved, sexual self.

Step 3: Ground and open

Put on all seven items of clothing. Perform whatever banishing and opening rituals are in your practice. Then find a comfortable position to ground, center, and shield. Feel into your body, maybe doing hip circles, or dancing, or stretching. You may sing or pray. Allow movement and your heart to guide you. At this point, invite any Goddesses,

Gods, guides, ascended masters, or other supportive beings into this ritual space. You may call on Inanna or another Goddess of glamour and beauty like Venus or Aphrodite. Ask for their guidance and compassion as they witness this process of sacred rebirth.

Step 4: Pass through the veils

Use the following script as a suggestion, allowing the moment, your heart, and your practice to guide you:

> *I stand before the Star, before the universe, before my own higher sexual self, embodied fully as* [Queen/King/Sovereign] *of Heaven and Earth. I stand in my beauty and power but must make my way to the underworld. I initiate this ritual of erotic embodiment, and death and rebirth, so I may be grounded in the powers of the flesh in this world and beyond.*

Remove your first piece of clothing. As you do this, feel a part of yourself being sacrificed. This is an intentional process of removal, of stripping away your human essence.

Say the following or adapt as you see fit:

> *I enter the first gate of the underworld and remove the sacred glamour of* [the item of clothing you're removing]. *As I shed this, so I shed* [your will/what this represents/what you're releasing].

Remove your second piece of clothing, and say:

> *I enter the second gate of the underworld and remove the sacred glamour of* [the item of clothing you're removing]. *As I shed this, so I shed* [your ego/what this represents/what you're releasing].

Remove your third piece of clothing, and say:

I enter the third gate of the underworld and remove the sacred glamour of [the item of clothing you're removing]. *As I shed this, so I shed* [your mental patterns/what this represents/what you're releasing].

Remove your fourth piece of clothing, and say:

I enter the fourth gate of the underworld and remove the sacred glamour of [the item of clothing you're removing]. *As I shed this, so I shed* [your concepts of my sacred sexuality/what this represents/ what you're releasing].

Remove your fifth piece of clothing, and say:

I enter the fifth gate of the underworld and remove the sacred glamour of [the item of clothing you're removing]. *As I shed this, so I shed* [your yearning for enlightenment/what this represents/what you're releasing].

Remove your sixth piece of clothing, and say:

I enter the sixth gate of the underworld and remove the sacred glamour of [the item of clothing you're removing]. *As I shed this, so I shed* [your lust of result with magick/what this represents/what you're releasing].

Remove your seventh and last piece of clothing, and say:

I enter the seventh and last gate of the underworld and remove the sacred glamour of [the item of clothing you're removing]. *As I shed this, so I shed* [your divinity/what this represents/what you're releasing].

Stand naked, feeling and embracing whatever comes up. Breathe into your body, running your hands over your bare flesh. How do you feel different? Take a moment to feel into whatever you're experiencing.

When you feel ready, say the following:

I stand in the underworld, in the darkness, in the void and abyss, completely naked. I stand here before the universe, bare and exposed, no longer of the Divine, but mortal. I stand here and allow myself to be sacrificed, so I may be reborn. So I may know who I am. So I may be totally and completely embodied in my erotic essence.

Step 5: Declaration of erotic embodiment

Now that you've found your way to beingness and humanness, it's time to step into your erotic power. Use the declaration of erotic embodiment you wrote before this ritual to make this quantum leap. Follow your heart, your vision, and your inner oracle as you say:

I stand upon the throne of the underworld, chthonic and cathartic, cleansed, stripped, and bared to the Gods. I stand embodied not in dress but in my flesh, spirit, and power. I stand here as a force and expression of the Divine Erotic, to declare myself an embodiment of this current. On this day, on all planes and all ways, I declare [your declaration of erotic embodiment]. *Through the darkness, I am re-born. I come back to myself and my flesh fully and completely, more grounded in my power than ever. I ascend as myself and more than myself, as a reflection of the sexual and carnal. This or something better for the highest good of all involved, as aligned with my True Will and purpose, so it is, and it is done.*

Stand here. You may meditate with the Star tarot card, feeling yourself as her, stripped bare but completely in your body. If you wish to carve a candle and anoint it for this working, do this now as well. Dwell here until you feel a shift, until you feel this declaration in your soul.

Step 6: Sex magick

Now you will be charging this declaration through sex magick. More than that, you will be connecting to your sexuality, to your body, and to pleasure in this new incarnation of self. This is beautiful and sensual and deep and special. Don't worry so much about orgasm or raising the energy as much as enjoying the experience. Melt into it. As you make self-love, be vulnerably present without any pressure. As you feel yourself getting ready to climax, or as close as you can, send this energy through the crown of your head to the universe to infuse your intention, *and also send this energy through your body so it feeds and nourishes you.* Stay in the afterglow as you breathe, visualizing yourself living your declaration of embodiment, and feeling this as truth.

Step 7: Ground and close

Find your way back to where you began. You may say something like the following to declare the ritual closed before you ground, shield, and close:

On all planes, in all ways, this working of death, rebirth, and erotic embodiment is complete. I come back from the underworld, transformed, and totally and completely me. I step into my flesh and sexual self fully and live from this place authentically. And so it is.

If you invited any Goddesses, Gods, spirit guides, or benevolent beings into the ritual, thank them and let them know the ritual is closed. Come back to yourself and your breath. Practice the closing rituals outlined earlier. Breathe, pressing your forehead into the ground like in a child's pose, sending any excess energy back into the earth. Practice banishing rituals, or clap, stomp your feet, laugh, chant, whoop, or yell one last time. Then record your ritual in your grimoire, exploring what's shifted. Drink water, eat something, and honor this new incarnation of self. If you carved a candle, let it burn all the way down if you can, leaving it in a sink, or snuffing or fanning it out. Relight it the next time you connect to your intention, and dispose of any wax at a garbage can at an intersection. And so it is.

NOW GO LIVE THE MAGICK OF THE DIVINE EROTIC

Well, beloved, you've reached the end of the book but the beginning of your journey. My hope is that you feel confident, capable, and inspired in connecting to your sexuality as a central part of your spiritual practice. My hope is that you are able to take the ritual and magick in this book and shape and shift them into something totally personal and resonant, your own brand of sacred sex that feels illuminating and subversive *for you*. My hope is that you feel self-assured in a new way, and that you're able to live a life embodied in sensual pleasures, devoted to whatever it is you believe in.

That's not to say that shame won't rear its ugly head or that this path will always be easy. But hopefully you now have more tools for how to deal with this than when you started. I know firsthand how life-changing it can be to connect with your sexuality as a part of a magickal path. I know how life-changing it can be to honor your sexuality as sacred, *as your own*. I hope that you've been able to taste this for yourself and have been able to experience the pleasures of the flesh not as sinful, but as divine and holy.

May the journey ahead be one filled with grace and connection, love, beauty, and ecstasy. May it help you find new paths to your heart, to love, to the world. May it be carnal and kinky and wild—but only if that's what you want! More than anything, may your journey with sacred sex through the path of the Divine Erotic be what your soul, mind, heart, and body need, on all planes, and in all ways, always. And so it is!

ACKNOWLEDGMENTS

I want to thank the Goddess for the opportunity to write this book. Babalon and Venus and Auset, thank you for your blessing, for this prayer and offering and devotional to the Divine Erotic in which you have entrusted me. I want to thank my incredible book editor, Nina Shield, for asking me to write this book. It means more than I have words for. And for my incredible agent, Jill Marr, for always having my back and believing in my work. To my teams at Sandra Dijkstra and TarcherPerigee, thank you, thank you, thank you. To my incredible family, my twin, Alexandra, and to my parents, Silvia and Ron, for always being there for me, for their unconditional love, and for their support. To my Tita, for all her support and blessings, to my Grandma Rose, for being my guide, to my Grandpas Harry and Jose, to all the angels in my family, and all the benevolent ancestors who have allowed me to be on this path. To Marissa, my star twin, for the never-ending support and laughs and bagels, and to Amelia, for our soulship and for being the best magickal partner one could ask for. To Goddess Daddy, for being the best sister in Divine Impurity I could ever imagine. To my friends, who have been there for me through this journey, and for always encouraging me to be bigger and badder, and not let shame make me shrink. To all my teachers in this realm and the astral, who have taught me, led me, guided me, and encouraged me. To Naha, for opening the door to Qabalah for me, to Alexandra Roxo, for being such a potent force in my exploration in the Divine Erotic, to all my exes and lovers, who reflected parts of myself to me that made this book possible to write. To my family at the Dominion, thank you for your unyielding inspiration, community, and love. To all the beloved interviewees who gave me the pleasure of knowledge and wisdom that I was able to infuse into this book. To the witches of the past, present, and future who have led me here and whose current I am deeply grateful to be a part of. To my occult muses and sex magicians of the past, to Los Angeles, to the faeries, to love, to sex, and the Divine Erotic. To the tarot, for being my muse, my guide, and my unyielding inspiration. To the Moon and Sun for their light, to the earth for her grounding wisdom, and the sky for its unyielding expanse. Thank you to the stars, from which I come and to where I return. And finally to the universe, for giving me this life.

NOTES

CHAPTER 1: INTO THE WORLD OF SACRED SEXUALITY

9 It is said—in gendered and dated terms—that through sexual union with his beloved: Urban, Hugh B. *Magia Sexualis: Sex, Magic, and Liberation in Modern Western Esotericism.* Berkeley: University of California Press, 2006.

10 Another example of eroticism in the Jewish scriptures is the Song of Songs: "Song of Songs 1." Sefaria. Accessed October 6, 2021. https://www.sefaria.org/Song_of_Songs.1.

10 Tantra, which most likely began in the first millennium CE: Gray, David B. "Tantra and the Tantric Traditions of Hinduism and Buddhism." *Oxford Research Encyclopedia of Religion*, April 5, 2016. Accessed September 7, 2021. https://oxfordre.com/religion/view/10.1093/acrefore/9780199340378.001.0001/acrefore-9780199340378-e-59.

10 you can think of it as "that which expands understanding": Feuerstein, Georg. *Sacred Sexuality: Living the Vision of the Erotic Spirit.* New York: J.P. Tarcher, 1992.

11 Tao makes up the invisible and visible world: Feuerstein. *Sacred Sexuality*, 1992.

11 Drawing or collecting chi into the body leads to transformation: Kenyon, Tom, and Judy Sion. *The Magdalen Manuscript: The Alchemies of Horus & the Sex Magic of Isis.* United States: ORB Communications, 2002.

11 This is done through practices like the microcosmic orbit: de Vos, Minke. *Tao Tantric Arts for Women: Cultivating Sexual Energy, Love, and Spirit.* Rochester, VT: Inner Traditions/Bear, 2016.

12 By cultivating a state of bliss and then contemplating that void: Kenyon and Sion. *The Magdalen Manuscript.* 2002.

12 **Gnosticism, like tantra, isn't a singular sect but many branches:** Urban. *Magia Sexualis*, 2006.

13 **You might have heard that Gnostics consumed sexual fluids and had orgies:** Urban. *Magia Sexualis*, 2006.

18 **In her potent, easy-to-read, and informative book *Come as You Are*, sex educator Emily Nagoski shares three messages:** Nagoski, Emily. *Come as You Are: The Surprising New Science That Will Transform Your Sex Life.* London: Simon & Schuster, 2015.

24 **These channels move through the etheric body:** Miller, Jason. *Sex, Sorcery, and Spirit: The Secrets of Erotic Magic.* United States: Red Wheel /Weiser, 2014.

36 **Alchemically, the Empress is salt, the body:** Miller. *Sex, Sorcery, and Spirit*, 2014.

CHAPTER 2: EXPANDING PLEASURE: SEX ED 101

61 **As of 2021, only thirty states:** Guttmacher Institute. "Sex and HIV Education," April 9, 2021. https://www.guttmacher.org/state-policy /explore/sex-and-hiv-education.

62 **And vulvas or pussies and penises or dicks:** Nagoski, Emily. *Come as You Are: The Surprising New Science That Will Transform Your Sex Life.* London: Simon & Schuster, 2015.

63 **If a hymen tears or bruises, it heals like any other part of the body:** Nagoski. *Come as You Are*, 2015.

64 **By lifting the pelvic floor, tightening the anus and perineum:** Miller, Jason. *Sex, Sorcery, and Spirit: The Secrets of Erotic Magic.* United States: Red Wheel/Weiser, 2014.

65 **The testicles begin to pull into the body:** Vernon, Betony. *The Boudoir Bible: The Uninhibited Sex Guide for Today.* New York: Rizzoli International Publications, Incorporated, 2013.

65 **Because the anatomy of those with vulvas is often ignored in scientific studies:** Engle, Gigi. *All the F*cking Mistakes: A Guide to Sex, Love, and Life.* New York: St. Martin's Publishing Group, 2020.

65 **The clitoris has two internal legs:** Salami, Minna. "This Is a 3D Model of a Clitoris—and the Start of a Sexual Revolution." *The Guardian*, September 15, 2016. https://www.theguardian.com/commentisfree/2016/sep/15 /3d-model-clitoris-sexual-revolution-sex-education-womens-sexuality.

65   **In total, the clitoris is composed of eighteen different parts:** Vernon. *The Boudoir Bible*, 2013.

66   **While those with penises have a 50 percent overlap between arousal:** Nagoski. *Come as You Are*, 2015.

66   **But arousal isn't just your body being aware of something sexual:** Nagoski. *Come as You Are*, 2015.

67   **In fact, sexual fantasies are so common:** "The Safest Sex," *Psychology Today*, June 9, 2016. https://www.psychologytoday.com/us/articles /199509/the-safest-sex#:~:text=Far%20from%20being%20a%20sign, fantasize%20least%2C%22%20Leitenberg%20notes.

67   **Science has recently shown:** "The Safest Sex." *Psychology Today*. 2016.

67   **Your fantasies also reflect your needs:** Lehmiller, Justin J. "The Deeper Psychological Meaning Behind Your Sex Fantasies." *Psychology Today*, July 3, 2018. https://www.psychologytoday.com/us/blog/the-myths-sex /201807/the-deeper-psychological-meaning-behind-your-sex-fantasies.

67   **You may have fantasies that are so intense they scare you:** Bivona, Jenny, and Joseph Critelli. "The Nature of Women's Rape Fantasies: An Analysis of Prevalence, Frequency, and Contents," *Journal of Sex Research*. U.S. National Library of Medicine, 2009. https://pubmed.ncbi.nlm.nih.gov /19085605/#:~:text=Results%20indicated%20that%2062%25%20 of,at%20least%20once%20a%20week.

68   **Thinking about and obsessing over orgasm is more likely to make you:** Nagoski. *Come as You Are*, 2015.

69   **The amount of dopamine released depends on context, culture, history:** "How Pleasure Affects Our Brains," *Neuroscience News*, April 29, 2018. https://neurosciencenews.com/pleasure-brain-8909/.

69   **That said, all experiences of pleasure are related to the same brain system:** Kringelbach, Morten L., and Kent C. Berridge. "The Neuroscience of Happiness and Pleasure." *Social Research*. U.S. National Library of Medicine, July 1, 2011. https://www.ncbi.nlm.nih.gov/pmc/articles /PMC3008658/.

77   **The Catholic Church defines lust as:** Catechism of the Catholic Church—The Sixth Commandment. Accessed April 27, 2021. https:// www.vatican.va/archive/ccc_css/archive/catechism/p3s2c2a6.htm.

CHAPTER 3: THE POWER OF SEX MAGICK

97 **While erotic spirituality has been around for thousands and thousands of years:** Urban, Hugh B. *Magia Sexualis: Sex, Magic, and Liberation in Modern Western Esotericism.* Berkeley: University of California Press, 2006.

97 **When he was born in 1875:** Urban. *Magia Sexualis,* 2006.

99 **Labeled an "erotic magical diabolist" and a "satanic occultist":** Urban. *Magia Sexualis,* 2006.

99 **He popularized a form of sigil-making that takes the letters:** Miller, Jason. *Sex, Sorcery, and Spirit: The Secrets of Erotic Magic.* Woodbury, MN: Red Wheel/Weiser, 2014.

99 **connected the concept of Divine light:** Kraig, Donald Michael. *Modern Sex Magick: Secrets of Erotic Spirituality.* Woodbury, MN: Llewellyn Publications, 2003.

100 **Fortune acted as a link between groups like the Ordo Templi Orientis (OTO) and the later pagan revival started:** Urban. *Magia Sexualis,* 2006.

100 **Eventually, she founded *de la Confrérie de la flèche d'or,* or the Brotherhood of the Golden Arrow:** Traxler, Donald, Hans Thomas Hakl, and Maria de Naglowska. *The Light of Sex: Initiation, Magic, and Sacrament.* Rochester, VT: Inner Traditions/Bear, 2011.

102 **With commercliazed sex decriminliazed, those in the industry can access:** Smith, Molly, and Juno Mac. *Revolting Prostitutes: The Fight for Sex Workers' Rights.* London: Verso, 2020.

103 **the exact history is disputed:** Budin, Stephanie Lynn. *The Myth of Sacred Prostitution in Antiquity.* Cambridge: Cambridge University Press, 2009.

CHAPTER 4: PREPARATION FOR THE PATH

138 **Like the mystic poets of the Sufis, like the Song of Solomon in the Bible:** Case, Paul Foster. *The Tarot: A Key to the Wisdom of the Ages.* New York: Jeremy P. Tarcher/Penguin, 2006.

CHAPTER 5: THE PATH OF ALCHEMY

157 **The Philosopher's Stone, which is the goal of alchemical work:** Bishop, Clifford. *Sex and Spirit: An Illustrated Guide to Sacred Sexuality.* Berkeley, CA: Ulysses Press, 2000.

157 **According to Paracelsus, the Philosopher's Stone is created through:** Bishop. *Sex and Spirit*, 2000.

160 **Originally, the sacred marriage was an erotic ritual of fertility:** Eisler, Riane. *Sacred Pleasure: Sex, Myth, and the Politics of the Body*. London: HarperCollins, 1995.

CHAPTER 6: THE PATH OF DIVINE UNION

178 **"Sex with soul is always a communion with another level of existence":** Moore, Thomas. *The Soul of Sex: Cultivating Life as an Act of Love*. New York: HarperCollins, 1999.

181 **The universe is a manifestation of play or polarization between Shakti and Shiva":** Feuerstein, Georg. *Tantra: The Path of Ecstasy*. Boston: Shambhala, 1998.

182 **The term originally referred to the "aspect of deity":** Patai, Raphael. *The Hebrew Goddess*. Detroit: Wayne State University Press, 1990.

183 **"Through love, we not only achieve unity with someone else":** Pollack, Rachel. *Seventy-Eight Degrees of Wisdom: A Tarot Journey to Self-Awareness* (a New Edition of the Tarot Classic). United States: Weiser Books, 2019.

CHAPTER 7: THE PATH OF THE MYSTIC

197 **These erotic votaries—or "sacred prostitutes":** Budin, Stephanie Lynn. *The Myth of Sacred Prostitution in Antiquity*. Cambridge: Cambridge University Press, 2009.

198 **This is where we get the term *Hierodule*:** Qualls-Corbett, Nancy. *The Sacred Prostitute: Eternal Aspect of the Feminine*. Toronto, Canada: Inner City Books, 1988.

199 **"Wherever the goddess of fertility, love, and passion was worshipped":** Qualls-Corbett. *The Sacred Prostitute*, 1988.

206 **As you already learned, the tantrikas:** Mumford, Jonn. *Ecstasy Through Tantra*. Woodbury, MN: Llewellyn Worldwide, Limited, 2021.

206 **Beyond this, tantric rituals are long and complex:** Mumford. *Ecstasy Through Tantra*, 2021.

CHAPTER 8: THE PATH OF THE DARK GOD/DESS

245 **Being kinky adds another layer:** Gerson, Merissa Nathan. "BDSM Versus the DSM," *The Atlantic.* January 14, 2015. https://www.theatlantic .com/health/archive/2015/01/bdsm-versus-the-dsm/384138/.

CHAPTER 10: THE PATH OF EROTIC EMBODIMENT

286 **In fact, glamour and fantasy go hand in hand:** Wilson, Robert Anton, and Grant Morrison. *Ishtar Rising: Why the Goddess Went to Hell and What to Expect Now That She's Returning.* Grand Junction, CO: Hilaritas Press, 2020.

303 **This ritual is inspired by the descent of the Sumerian Goddess Inanna:** Kramer, Samuel Noah, Elizabeth Williams-Forte, and Diane Wolkstein. *Inanna.* New York: HarperCollins, 1983.

RESOURCES

In this section I share some resources to help you along your sacred sex journey. You will find a list of all the wonderful souls I interviewed for this book, including sex workers, sexuality professionals, kink-informed therapists, and more. You also will find links to my favorite sex toy stores, resources to support the decriminalization of sex work, a list of erotic tarot decks to work with, and resources for learning about kink. My hope is that this section helps you continue on your dance with the Divine Erotic by reminding you that you're not alone on this journey. I see you, I love you, and you got this.

INTERVIEWEES FOR THIS BOOK

HAVEN AND SEBASTIAN

Haven is a lover of love, aspiring writer, and adventurer. She works in the human services industry. She has built a life and career around human connection while advocating for those who face hardship and marginalization. She is a partner, mother, daughter, sister, and friend.

Sebastian tries to find balance between being a husband, dad, executive, athlete, and resident of the place where philosophy and physics meet. When he isn't at home, you can find him in the ocean or on a trail.

SYDNEY JONES

Sydney Jones is a clinical hypnotherapist, professional dominatrix, published author, and intuitive psychic residing in Southern California. Sydney uses her decades of experience to help her clients embrace their sexuality and personal power through healing shadow work, hypnotherapy, and radical self-love. She believes incorporating sex magic into healing work can greatly increase someone's ability to break through their barriers to claiming their power in a unique and potent way. Sydney received her bachelor's degree in women's studies and religious studies from San Diego State University and her master's degree in creative writing from National University.

Find Sydney at:
www.goddesssydney.com

Connect with her at:
Instagram / TikTok: @goddessunveiledtarot

LINA DUNE

Lina Dune is a bisexual submissive in a 24/7 D/s relationship and a proponent of sane and healing BDSM. She goes by @askasub on Instagram, where she makes kink-centered memes, gives D/s relationship advice, and serves as fairy-submother to all who seek her advice. She is also the host and creator of the *Ask a Sub* podcast, where she answers D/s relationship questions with her trademark warmth and wit.

Find Lina at:
www.askasub.com

Connect with her at:
Instagram / Twitter: @askasub. You can find her podcast on Apple and Spotify.

AMELIA QUINT

Amelia Quint brings a decade of experience as a professional astrologer and witch. Her writings and work in the sacred arts have been featured in *Allure*, *Teen Vogue*, *Glamour*, *Nylon*, and many others. She is also the resident astrology expert for the Bumble app. Amelia hosts the *Bad Astrologers* podcast and is available for readings and mentoring. Her work is LGBTQIA+ affirming, polyamory positive, and kink friendly. She believes in cocreating your life with the stars and is on a mission to make astrology more fun, positive, and magical.

Find Amelia at:
www.ameliaquint.com

Connect with her at:
Instagram: @ameliaquint_ / Twitter: @ameliaquint

STEFANI GOERLICH

Stefani Goerlich is a certified sex therapist and author of the award-winning book *The Leather Couch: Clinical Practice with Kinky Clients*. She owns and operates Bound Together Counseling, where she specializes in working with religious minorities as well as gender, sexuality, and relationship diversities.

Connect with her at:
www.boundtogethercounseling.com

Her book:
The Leather Couch: Clinical Practice with Kinky Clients

RYUN HARRISON

Ryun Harrison is a creative by day and a mystic 24/7. His love of all things *materia magica* has led him down a path toward a more unified and balanced relationship with the Divine. The Abyss Tarot is the result of his connection to tarot, channeled collage, and the gay experience. Ryun lives by the western waters of NYC. Follow him down the Abyss, and find yourself again . . .

Find The Abyss Tarot at:
www.theabysstarot.com

Connect with Ryun at:
Instagram: @baebae_yaga or @theabysstarot

DOMINA DIA DYNASTY

Dia Dynasty is a *shamanatrix*, a professional dominatrix who incorporates spiritual and ritual modalities into her BDSM practice in order to offer her clients transformational and life-altering experiences. Her twelve years as a pro domme in New York City and worldwide, alongside her lifelong engagement with yoga, magick, and metaphysics, have honed Dia's skills of healing with a mixture of witchcraft, energy work, holistic health practices, and bespoke rituals. She has a familiar named Lady and is the Matriarch of the Femdom Farm, an upstate New York kink retreat.

Find Domina Dia at:
www.dominadynasty.com

Connect with her at:
Instagram: @dia__dynasty / Twitter: @DominaDynasty

ISABELLA FRAPPIER

Isabella Frappier is a sexual activist and pleasure mentor focused on body literacy and sexual sovereignty. Isabella works with clients in one-on-one video sessions and in group workshops such as Eros Community to help them embrace their sexuality, incorporating aspects of feminist BDSM, sex magic, and even astrology into her work. She is also a host on the popular *Sex Magic* podcast.

Find Isabella at:
www.isabellafrappier.com

Connect with her on:
Instagram: @bellatookaphoto / Twitter: @RiseOfAphrodite

PAM SHAFFER, LMFT

Pam Shaffer is a licensed marriage and family psychotherapist and founder of Best Self Psych and Galaxy Brains, where she provides individual and couples therapy for California residents and coaching online worldwide. She's a compassionate guide who helps others through the ups and downs of life with pragmatism and a bit of magick. Her practice is ENM, kink, and LGBTQIA + affirmative. She mainly helps people who are experiencing difficulty in their relationships and professional and creative lives, and her specialties include working with the effects of depression, anxiety, C-PTSD, and ADHD. As a musician, podcast host, clinician, and recovered manic pixie dream girl, Pam brings a creative and multifaceted collaborative approach to all she does.

Connect with Pam at:
www.bestselfpsych.com

STORES

Babeland Toy Store
www.babeland.com
@babeland_toys

The Pleasure Chest
www.thepleasurechest.com

The Smitten Kitten
www.smittenkittenonline.com

The Stockroom
www.stockroom.com

EROTIC TAROT AND ORACLE DECKS

Eros Garden of Love Tarot
Slutist Tarot
Manara Tarot
Manara Erotic Oracle

Tarot of Sexual Magic
Decameron Tarot
Kamasutra Tarot
Erotic Fantasy Tarot
Valentina Tarot
Tantric Dakini Oracle

BEGINNER BDSM BOOKS

SM 101 by Jay Wiseman
Screw the Roses, Send Me the Thorns by Phillip Miller and Molly Devon
The Ultimate Guide to Kink by Tristan Toaramino
The New Bottoming Book by Dossie Easton and Janet W. Hardy
The New Topping Book by Dossie Easton and Janet W. Hardy

SEX WORKER ADVOCACY
AND MUTUAL AID GROUPS

SWOP (Sex Worker Outreach Project) USA
www.swopusa.org

SWARM (Sex Worker Advocacy and Resistance Movement) Collective
www.swarmcollective.org

St James Infirmary
www.stjamesinfirmary.org

Red Canary Song
www.redcanarysong.net

Black Sex Worker Collective
www.blacksexworkercollective.org

Sex Workers Project
www.sexworkersproject.org

Desiree Alliance
www.desireealliance.org

KINK RESOURCES

Shibari Study
www.shibaristudy.com

Kink Coven
www.kinkcoven.love

Midori
www.fhp-inc.com/resources/

The Twisted Monk
https://www.twistedmonk.com
https://www.youtube.com/user
/twistedmonkstudios

Vox Body
www.voxbody.com

SEX ED RESOURCES

Haylin Belay, sex educator and pleasure witch
https://www.haylin.co
https://www.haylin.co/sexedforall

BIBLIOGRAPHY

"Apollo." Encyclopædia Britannica. Accessed July 31, 2021. https://www
.britannica.com/topic/Apollo-Greek-mythology.

Auryn, Mat. *Psychic Witch: A Metaphysical Guide to Meditation, Magick &
Manifestation*. Woodbury, MN: Llewellyn Worldwide, Limited, 2020.

Berrett-Ibarria, Sofia. "Sex Workers Pioneered the Early Internet—and It
Screwed Them Over," VICE, 2018. https://www.vice.com/en/article
/qvazy7/sex-workers-pioneered-the-early-internet.

Bishop, Clifford. *Sex and Spirit: An Illustrated Guide to Sacred Sexuality*. Berkeley, CA: Ulysses Press, 2000.

Bivona, Jenny, and Joseph Critelli. "The Nature of Women's Rape Fantasies:
An Analysis of Prevalence, Frequency, and Contents," *Journal of Sex Research*. U.S. National Library of Medicine, 2009. https://pubmed.ncbi
.nlm.nih.gov/19085605/#:~:text=Results%20indicated%20that%2062
%25%20of,at%20least%20once%20a%20week.

Budin, Stephanie Lynn. *The Myth of Sacred Prostitution in Antiquity*. Cambridge: Cambridge University Press, 2009.

Case, Paul Foster. *The Tarot: A Key to the Wisdom of the Ages*. New York: Jeremy
P. Tarcher/Penguin, 2006.

Cashford, Jules, and Anne Baring. *The Myth of the Goddess: Evolution of an
Image*. London: Penguin Books Limited, 1993.

Catechism of the Catholic Church—The Sixth Commandment. Accessed
April 27, 2021. https://www.vatican.va/archive/ccc_css/archive/catechism
/p3s2c2a6.htm.

de Vos, Minke. *Tao Tantric Arts for Women: Cultivating Sexual Energy, Love,
and Spirit*. Rochester, VT: Inner Traditions/Bear, 2016.

Duquette, Lon Milo. *Understanding Aleister Crowley's Thoth Tarot*. United States: Weiser Books, 2003.

Eisler, Riane. *Sacred Pleasure: Sex, Myth, and the Politics of the Body*. London: HarperCollins, 1995.

Ember, Carol R., and Christina Carolus. "Altered States of Consciousness," Explaining Human Culture. Human Relations Area Files, January 10, 2017. https://hraf.yale.edu/ehc/summaries/altered-states-of-consciousness.

Engle, Gigi. *All the F*cking Mistakes: A Guide to Sex, Love, and Life*. New York: St. Martin's Publishing Group, 2020.

Feuerstein, Georg. *Sacred Sexuality: Living the Vision of the Erotic Spirit*. New York: J.P. Tarcher, 1992.

Geczy, Adam, and Vicki Karaminas. *Libertine Fashion: Sexual Freedom, Rebellion, and Style*. London: Bloomsbury Academic, 2020.

Gerson, Merissa Nathan. "BDSM Versus the DSM," *The Atlantic*. January 14, 2015. https://www.theatlantic.com/health/archive/2015/01/bdsm-versus-the-dsm/384138/.

Gray, David B. "Tantra and the Tantric Traditions of Hinduism and Buddhism," *Oxford Research Encyclopedia of Religion*, April 5, 2016. Accessed September 7, 2021. https://oxfordre.com/religion/view/10.1093/acrefore/9780199340378.001.0001/acrefore-9780199340378-e-59.

Griffin, Susan. *The Book of the Courtesans: A Catalogue of Their Virtues*. New York: Broadway Books, 2002.

Guttmacher Institute. "Sex and HIV Education," April 9, 2021. https://www.guttmacher.org/state-policy/explore/sex-and-hiv-education.

Herstik, Gabriela. "Whipping the Brain: The Mind-Altering, Hallucinatory States of BDSM," *MEL Magazine*, March 13, 2020. https://melmagazine.com/en-us/story/whipping-the-brain-the-mind-altering-hallucinatory-states-of-bdsm.

History.com Editors. "Buddhism." History.com. A&E Television Networks, October 12, 2017. https://www.history.com/topics/religion/buddhism.

"How Pleasure Affects Our Brains," *Neuroscience News*, April 29, 2018. https://neurosciencenews.com/pleasure-brain-8909/.

Kenyon, Tom, and Judy Sion. *The Magdalen Manuscript: The Alchemies of Horus & the Sex Magic of Isis*. United States: ORB Communications, 2002.

Kingsland, James. "Sleep, Drugs and Mental Health: How Altered States of Consciousness Could Keep Us Happy," *BBC Science Focus Magazine*, November 19, 2019. https://www.sciencefocus.com/the-human-body/sleep -drugs-and-mental-health-how-altered-states-of-consciousness-could -keep-us-happy/.

Kraig, Donald Michael. *Modern Sex Magick: Secrets of Erotic Spirituality.* Woodbury, MN: Llewellyn Publications, 2003.

Kramer, Samuel Noah, Elizabeth Williams-Forte, and Diane Wolkstein. *Inanna.* New York: HarperCollins, 1983.

Kringelbach, Morten L., and Kent C. Berridge. "The Neuroscience of Happiness and Pleasure," *Social Research.* U.S. National Library of Medicine, July 1, 2011. https://www.ncbi.nlm.nih.gov/pmc/articles/PMC3008658/.

Lehmiller, Justin J. "The Deeper Psychological Meaning Behind Your Sex Fantasies," *Psychology Today*, July 3, 2018. https://www.psychologytoday .com/us/blog/the-myths-sex/201807/the-deeper-psychological-meaning -behind-your-sex-fantasies.

Miller, Jason. *Sex, Sorcery, and Spirit: The Secrets of Erotic Magic.* United States: Red Wheel/Weiser, 2014.

Moore, Thomas. *The Soul of Sex: Cultivating Life as an Act of Love.* New York: HarperCollins, 1999.

Mumford, Jonn. *Ecstasy Through Tantra.* Woodbury, MN: Llewellyn Publications, 2021.

Nagoski, Emily. *Come as You Are: The Surprising New Science That Will Transform Your Sex Life.* London: Simon & Schuster, 2015.

Paris, Ginette. *Pagan Grace: Dionysus, Hermes and Goddess Memory.* Ashland, OH: Spring 1990.

Patai, Raphael. *The Hebrew Goddess.* Detroit: Wayne State University Press, 1990.

Petronis, Lexi. "13 Benefits of Orgasms We Could All Use Right Now," *Glamour*, December 13, 2013. https://www.glamour.com/story /6-super-surprising-health-bene.

Pollack, Rachel. *Seventy-Eight Degrees of Wisdom: A Book of Tarot.* United States: Weiser Books, 2009.

Qualls-Corbett, Nancy. *The Sacred Prostitute: Eternal Aspect of the Feminine.* Toronto, Canada: Inner City Books, 1988.

Radcliffe, Shawn. "Lovemaking and Altered States of Consciousness," Science and Nonduality. Accessed May 24, 2021. https://www.science andnonduality.com/article/lovemaking-and-altered-states-of-con sciousness.

Regardie, Israel. *The Philosopher's Stone: Spiritual Alchemy, Psychology, and Ritual Magic.* Woodbury, MN: Llewellyn Publications, 2013.

———. *The Tree of Life: A Study in Magic.* United States: S. Weiser, 1972.

"The Safest Sex." *Psychology Today,* June 9, 2016. https://www.psychologyto day.com/us/articles/199509/the-safest-sex#:~:text=Far%20from%20be ing%20a%20sign,fantasize%20least%2C%22%20Leitenberg%20 notes.

Salami, Minna. "This Is a 3D Model of a Clitoris—and the Start of a Sexual Revolution," *The Guardian,* September 15, 2016. https://www.theguard ian.com/commentisfree/2016/sep/15/3d-model-clitoris-sexual-revolution -sex-education-womens-sexuality.

Schreck, Nikolas, and Zeena Schreck. *Demons of the Flesh: The Complete Guide to Left Hand Path Sex Magic.* United Kingdom: Creation Books, 2002.

Smith, Molly, and Juno Mac. *Revolting Prostitutes: The Fight for Sex Workers' Rights.* London: Verso, 2020.

Smith, Patti. *Just Kids.* London: Bloomsbury, 2011.

"Song of Songs 1." Sefaria. Accessed October 6, 2021. https://www.sefaria .org/Song_of_Songs.1.

"Techniques for Inducing Mystical Experiences." Encyclopædia Britannica. Accessed May 26, 2021. https://www.britannica.com/topic/mysticism /Techniques-for-inducing-mystical-experiences.

Traxler, Donald, Hans Thomas Hakl, and Maria de Naglowska. *The Light of Sex: Initiation, Magic, and Sacrament.* Rochester, VT: Inner Traditions/ Bear, 2011.

Urban, Hugh B. *Magia Sexualis: Sex, Magic, and Liberation in Modern Western Esotericism.* Berkeley: University of California Press, 2006.

Vernon, Betony. *The Boudoir Bible: The Uninhibited Sex Guide for Today.* New York: Rizzoli International Publications, Incorporated, 2013.

Walker, Barbara G. *The Woman's Encyclopedia of Myths and Secrets.* New York: Harper & Row, 1983.

Wang, Robert. *The Qabalistic Tarot: A Textbook of Mystical Philosophy.* United States: Red Wheel/Weiser, 1987.

Wilson, Robert Anton, and Grant Morrison. *Ishtar Rising: Why the Goddess Went to Hell and What to Expect Now That She's Returning.* Grand Junction, CO: Hilaritas Press, 2020.

Gabriela Herstik is the author of *Inner Witch: A Modern Guide to the Ancient Craft*, *Bewitching the Elements: A Guide to Empowering Yourself Through Earth, Air, Fire, Water, and Spirit*, and *Embody Your Magick: A Guided Journal for the Modern Witch*. She has written for outlets such as *VOGUE International*, *Glamour*, *i-D*, *Cosmopolitan*, and *Dazed Beauty* on witchcraft and magick and has headed columns for *NYLON*, *High Times*, and *Chakrubs* on the intersection of glamour, sexuality, and the Feminine Divine. She has been featured in publications around the world such as *The Guardian*, *LA Weekly*, *Tattler Asia*, *The Atlantic*, *USA Weekly*, and *VOGUE Spain* on her contribution to the occult milieu. Gabriela has been a practicing witch since the tender age of thirteen, and is a devotee of the Goddess of Love and Lust. Gabriela leads kinky rituals and discussion circles, writes ritual guides for the lunations and holidays of the Witch, and creates erotic art inspired by the power and magick of the flesh. She believes magick is for everyone. You can keep up with her at gabrielaherstik.com and on Instagram and Twitter at @gabyherstik.